"How did this happen?"

A practical guide to understanding eating disorders

TABLE of CONTENTS

Chapter 7: Treating Eating Disorders

Chapter 8: Seeking Additional Help

Foreword

This book is dedicated to all of the courageous people who have come together to fight the battle against eating disorders. Already, too many men and women have endured the pain and suffering that eating disorders inflict upon a person's life. Families and loved ones often suffer in silence as the person they care about seems to change—both physically and emotionally—before their very eyes. Almost instinctively, they will ask, *"How did this happen?"* Implicit in this question are feelings of blame, shame and guilt. This book was written to address how eating disorders do happen—and to help the reader understand that "the person is not the problem; the problem is the problem." No one person or thing has caused these life-altering disorders.

Even though no one is to blame, loved ones often remain baffled by what to do and are burdened by feelings of helplessness and doubt. In particular, they may wonder whether the eating disorder battle will ever be won. This book addresses those feelings head-on. In every chapter, you will find the strong message that eating disorders can be conquered.

In creating this book, we wanted to equip the reader with a basic overview of all the information necessary to address the problem of eating disorders. Therefore, this book covers all of the areas that you may have questions or concerns about—including preventing, identifying and treating eating disorders, getting help for someone you know who may have an eating disorder, and what to expect if formal treatment is necessary. Because the multidisciplinary approach to treatment is one of the most effective methods of treating these disorders, we enlisted the help of many experts to make this book the most comprehensive, accurate, and useful resource possible. Our review panel included physicians, physical and occupational therapists, registered nurses, psychiatrists, psychologists, dietitians, and health educators.

The front cover of this book is illustrative of the long path to recovery that many patients must follow in order to get back their lives and dreams. Indeed, the journey is a series of small steps, unexpected setbacks, rocky obstacles, and of course, huge leaps forward. Whether you are just hoping to learn more about eating disorders or are facing one right now, we hope that this book can be both your boots and your compass—a resource that makes the trail more bearable, and a tool that reliably points you in the right direction.

CHAPTER 1

Understanding Eating Disorders

Introduction

You stand for a moment in a crowd and carefully observe all of those around you. You see individuals of various ages with different body shapes and sizes. The differences in their physical characteristics may be obvious, and you might even think that someone has a problem with being overweight or underweight. You begin to compare your own physical characteristics with some of these individuals. However, although disheartened by your own weight issues and your inability to modify your habits, you shrug your shoulders and move on, vowing to start a diet or exercise program another day because you're simply too tired or too busy to do it now.

Contrast your own thoughts under these circumstances with people who have been struggling with an eating disorder. They may obsess about their weight, frequently comparing themselves to others and often spending up to 100 percent of their day thinking about weight, body image, food and exercise. The rules of the eating disorder may require that they weigh themselves more than 20 times a day. They may feel driven to engage in dramatic binges, in which huge quantities of food are consumed in a short time and may or may not be followed by self-induced purging by vomiting. Characteristic of this behavior is a sense of total lack of control. Some people who have an eating disorder become increasingly isolated, shunning food to the point where they feel bloated and horribly uncomfortable from eating so much as a simple salad or bowl of soup.

Many individuals with eating disorders are at a normal weight or even overweight; others are extremely underweight yet see themselves as hopelessly fat and unattractive. Depression, anxiety, compulsions and addictions can intensify these feelings. Despite being tortured by eating disorders, people can maintain what looks like a normal lifestyle—at least on the outside. However, should an eating disorder continue, it can lead to physical deprivation, emotional turmoil, guilt and fear.

In many cases, eating disorders first appear when people try to live a healthier lifestyle by cutting fat out of their meals or by exercising more. However, some of the changes can become unhealthy when they lead to serious obsessions. Dieting sometimes leads to weight loss but may also lead to extreme hunger that, in turn, can lead to overeating. An intense fear of gaining weight may then result in the individual beginning to binge and purge in an effort to eat without gaining weight. Individuals also may attempt to compensate for eating by increasing their exercise, sometimes to levels that cause weight loss.

Eating disorders—which include anorexia nervosa, bulimia nervosa, eating disorder not otherwise specified and binge-eating disorder—clearly involve the complex interaction of physical and emotional issues. In addition, eating disorders may coexist with depression, anxiety, compulsions and addictions.

Some facts about eating disorders

It is estimated that eating disorders occur in 1 to 10 percent of the population with even higher rates being reported in certain subgroups such as dancers, models, actresses and athletes. Our ability to prevent the development of eating disorders in the general population is hampered by our limited understanding of the risk factors that may influence the development of eating disorders.

Eating disorders are widespread among adolescents. One school-based study found that 11 percent of 15-year-old girls vomited to control weight, 8 percent used diet pills and 7 percent used laxatives. Here are some additional facts:

- One study indicated that 80 percent of girls reported they had already been on a diet to lose weight before the age of 13.
- Research suggests that about 4 percent of college-aged women have bulimia.
- About 5 to 10 percent of people with anorexia and bulimia are male.
- Anorexia and bulimia affect people primarily in their teens and twenties, but there have been reports of both disorders in children as young as 6 and individuals as old as 76.
- One study of 695 male and female athletes found many examples of bulimia nervosa attitudes and behavior. A third of the group was preoccupied with food. About 25 percent binge-ate at least once a week. Over 15 percent thought they were overweight when they were not. About 12 percent feared losing control, or actually did lose control, when they ate. More than 5 percent ate until they were gorged and nauseated.
- A research project done by the National Collegiate Athletic Association (NCAA) looked at the number of student athletes who experienced an eating disorder in the previous two years. Over 93 percent of the reported problems were in women's sports. The sports that had the highest number of participants

with eating disorders, in descending order, were women's cross country, women's gymnastics, women's swimming, and women's track and field events.

SOURCES:

Anorexia Nervosa and Related Eating Disorders, Inc. (ANRED)

Taylor, CB et al. Factors associated with weight concerns in adolescent girls. Eating Disorders 24(1); 31-42.

Johnson, C.; Powers, PS.; Dick, R. Athletes and eating disorders: the National Collegiate Athletic Association study. International Journal of Eating Disorders 1999 Sep; 26(2); 179-188.

How is an eating disorder diagnosed?

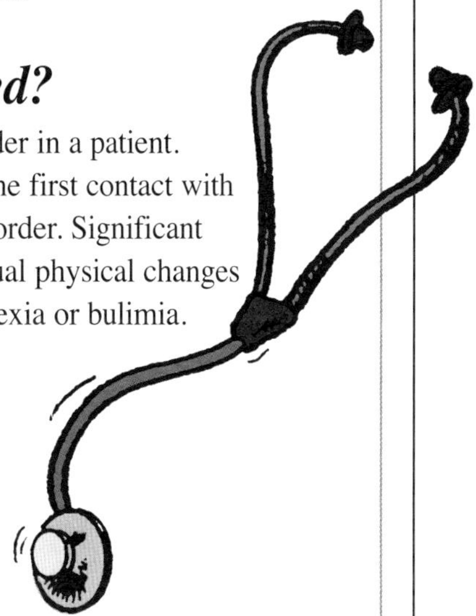

Primary care physicians can initially detect an eating disorder in a patient. Family physicians, pediatricians and internists often have the first contact with patients who may be displaying symptoms of an eating disorder. Significant fluctuations in a patient's weight and the detection of unusual physical changes can alert the physician to the possible development of anorexia or bulimia. To determine if an eating disorder is present, a health care provider may ask some of the following questions:

- Do you count calories and fat grams every time you eat or drink?
- Do you constantly think about food, weight or body image?
- Do you vomit after eating or use laxatives or diuretics to keep your weight down?
- Do you determine your mood for the entire day based on the number on your scale?
- Do you exercise because you have to, not because you want to?

Answers to these questions, along with a physical exam, help a doctor determine if further evaluation is necessary. He or she may contact an eating disorder clinic for further consultation. A patient may be hospitalized when the patient is considered medically compromised (e.g., has low blood pressure, low body temperature, or physical symptoms such as chest pain) and is in need of 24-hour medical attention. The medical data that the primary physician collects is critical for initiating the admissions process.

In most cases when a primary care physician consults an eating disorder program, the recommendation will be for the patient to have an initial assessment. (For more information on assessments, please see page 48.)

The actual diagnosis of an eating disorder involves a number of different criteria. In some cases, symptoms meet the criteria for a diagnosis of anorexia nervosa; other times, the diagnosis will be bulimia nervosa or binge-eating disorder. In some situations, a patient may not meet the criteria for either bulimia or anorexia, yet an eating disorder still exists. In such cases, the eating disorder is actually called "eating disorder not otherwise specified." This diagnosis is as serious as anorexia and bulimia.

A number of tools are available to help doctors and therapists determine if someone has an eating disorder. Many individuals with significant eating issues may not meet all the specific criteria; however, they still need an assessment. One standard tool is the Diagnostic and Statistical Manual of Mental Disorders (DSM-IV). Published in 1994, it lists behaviors that may specify the presence of an eating disorder. The specific criteria for eating disorders appear in the shaded boxes on pages 7–10.

Medical problems associated with eating disorders

Poor nutrition caused by some eating disorders can lead to many medical problems. These problems can affect just about every system in the body. It is important that people with eating disorders keep in close contact with their primary care providers and alert them to any medical problems they may be experiencing. The following are just a few of the problems most often found.

Heart and Blood Vessels

A number of serious effects of poor nutrition and dehydration involve the heart and blood vessels. The heart can actually lose up to 25 percent of its muscle and become less efficient at pumping. Sometimes this deterioration can lead to chest pain and shortness of breath. It can also cause dizziness and fainting, particularly if daily fluid intake is inadequate. People with eating disorders, for instance, may notice dizziness when they get up suddenly from lying down or sitting. In addition, excessive exercise can affect the nerves that control the heart rate, often causing the heart rate to slow to 40 beats a minute or less. Although many people think that a low heart rate is a healthy sign (since some marathon runners have slow heart rates), it often is not. In fact, exercise coupled with poor nutrition or dehydration can place serious stress on the heart. Diet pills and water pills, or even a high caffeine intake, can add to this stress by increasing the work required of the heart. Dehydration lowers the amount of fluid volume in the blood vessels and can cause dangerous reductions in the blood pressure, which is required for all body functions. When the blood pressure falls too much, there is not enough pressure to send blood to the brain, so fainting and black-out spells may occur.

Stomach and Intestines

The stomach and intestines (or "bowel") require lots of nerve and blood vessel interactions to work properly. Therefore, those things that affect the heart and blood vessels also affect the stomach and intestines. In addition, people who use laxatives excessively lose additional fluids, and their bowel becomes so accustomed to the laxatives that it doesn't want to function without them. When the bowel doesn't function properly or laxatives are discontinued, fluid retention occurs, and the cycle continues. With a very restrictive diet, the stomach actually shrinks, causing a false sense of fullness when normal quantities of food are eaten. For those individuals who purge frequently, the esophagus (food tube that goes from the throat to the stomach) becomes very irritated from stomach acid constantly coming up. This irritation can cause bleeding or in the most serious cases, rupture of the esophagus or stomach from continued vomiting. Sometimes individuals develop acid reflux, in which the stomach acid simply begins to come up without the individual even trying to purge. This continuous reflux can also cause irritation of the stomach and esophagus. Finally, both purging and acid reflux can cause one of the most serious complications: An individual may accidentally inhale stomach acid into the lungs, which can be fatal.

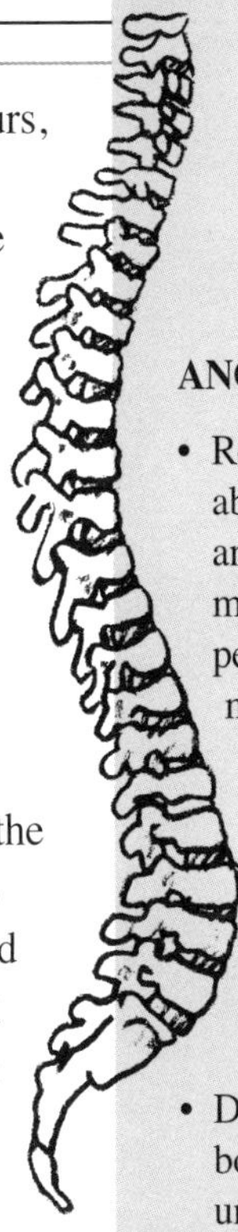

Bones

When eating disorders cause vitamin and calcium deficiency, osteoporosis can occur. Osteoporosis, the medical name for thin bones, can lead to a susceptibility for developing bone fractures. During the early years, when a person is growing, the bone that is developed will determine the strength of the bones well into adulthood. The stronger one's bones are in youth, the healthier the bones will be as the body ages. We cannot increase our bone density after the age of 30, but we can continue to build it up until that age.

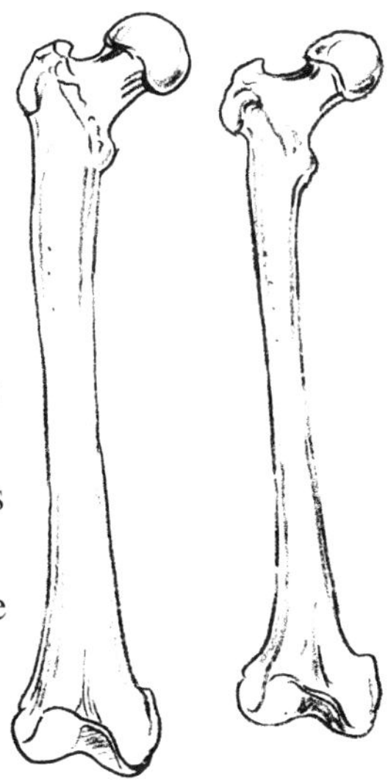

Normal healthy femur compared to a femur stunted by an eating disorder

DSM-IV Criteria for Types of Eating Disorders

ANOREXIA NERVOSA

- Refusal to maintain body weight at or above a minimally normal weight for age and height (weight loss leading to maintenance of body weight less than 85 percent of that expected; or failure to make expected weight gain during period of growth, leading to body weight less than 85 percent of that expected)
- Intense fear of gaining weight or becoming fat, even though underweight
- Disturbance in the way in which one's body weight or shape is experienced, undue influence of body weight or shape on self-evaluation, or denial of the seriousness of the current low body weight
- In postmenarcheal females, amenorrhea—the absence of at least three consecutive menstrual cycles. (A woman is considered to have lost her menstrual periods if her periods occur only following hormone administration.)

Type I: Restricting Subtype

During the current episode of anorexia nervosa, the person has not regularly engaged in binge-eating or purging behavior (i.e., self-induced vomiting or the misuse of laxatives, diuretics or enemas)

Type II: Binge-Eating/Purging Subtype

During the current episode of anorexia nervosa, the person has regularly engaged in binge-eating or purging behavior (i.e., self-induced vomiting or the misuse of laxatives, diuretics or enemas.)

DSM-IV Criteria for Eating Disorders (cont.)

BULIMIA NERVOSA

- Recurrent episodes of binge-eating. An episode of binge-eating is characterized by both of the following:
  - —Eating, in a discrete period of time (e.g., within any 2-hour period), an amount of food that is definitely larger than most people would eat during a similar period of time and under similar circumstances
  - —A sense of lack of control over eating during the episode (e.g., a feeling that one cannot stop eating or control what or how much one is eating)
- Recurrent inappropriate compensatory behavior in order to prevent weight gain, such as self-induced vomiting; misuse of laxatives, diuretics, enemas, or other medications; fasting; or excessive exercise
- Binge-eating and inappropriate compensatory behaviors that occur, on average, at least twice a week for 3 months
- Self-evaluation unduly influenced by body shape and weight
- The disturbance does not occur exclusively during episodes of bulimia nervosa.

Type I: Restricting Subtype

Purging Type: During the current episode of bulimia nervosa, the person has regularly engaged in self-induced vomiting or the misuse of laxatives, diuretics, or enemas.

Type II: Nonpurging Type

During the current episode of bulimia nervosa, the person has used other inappropriate compensatory behaviors, such as fasting or excessive exercise, but has not regularly engaged in self-induced vomiting or the misuse of laxatives, diuretics, or enemas.

Reproductive organs

Many women with eating disorders lose their menstrual period because of low hormone levels from inadequate nutrition with weight loss or excessive exercising. Lowered hormone levels can also cause thinning of the bones and a reduced sex drive. Males with eating disorders also are affected by a reduction in male hormones, which can lead to a lower sex drive and reduced sexual functioning. Both men and women also experience actual physical changes in the reproductive organs from excessive weight loss. In women, the size of the ovaries is decreased, the uterus itself becomes smaller and the lining of the vagina can become dry and irritated, causing pain with intercourse. In men, eating disorders can decrease the size of the testicles. Finally, fertility can be reduced in both men and women.

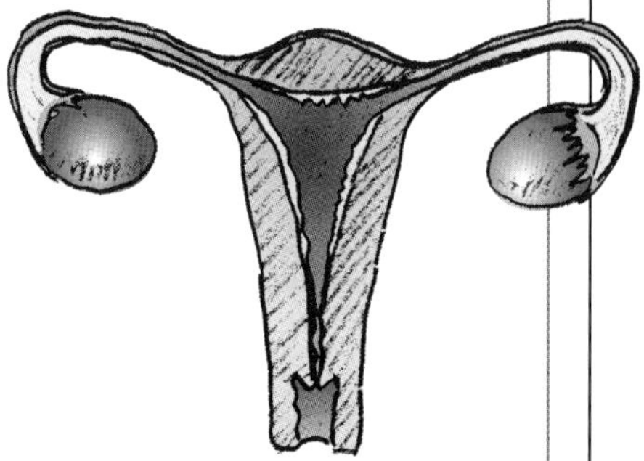

Teeth and mouth health

Dental hygiene is of concern for those with eating disorders because of the risk for vitamin deficiencies and gum disorder as well as cavities for those who purge regularly. With purging, in fact, the enamel on the teeth can be permanently eroded and discolored. The use of the finger to induce vomiting can cause bumps on the fingers which grow in response to constant scraping of the finger against the teeth. Sometimes the finger or whatever is used to induce vomiting can scrape the mouth area and cause bleeding.

Are medications used to treat eating disorders?

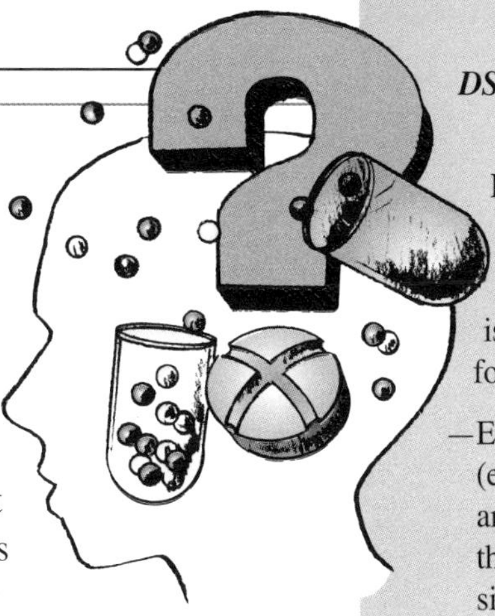

Although the treatment of medical problems frequently involves the use of medications, it is important to know that this is not always true in the treatment of eating disorders. However, under certain circumstances, particularly when eating disorders are associated with depression, anxiety, obsessive ideas or compulsive behaviors, anti-depressant or anti-anxiety medication may very well be beneficial. Sometimes, medications can allow the individual to better focus on fighting the eating disorder itself. In other cases where binge-eating and purging is a prominent feature, anti-depressant medication has been shown to help quiet the thoughts and behaviors. However, it is important to keep in mind that anti-depressant medication can take several weeks to reach its full effect.

Poor nutrition can lead to a slowing of the thinking process and symptoms that mimic depression. Thus, it may be necessary for individuals to regain some weight before medications can be considered. In many cases, the individual's mood and thinking process will quickly improve with better nutrition. In other cases, it will become more clear as to whether medication is needed and which medications are indicated.

Medications can be life saving or even simply make treatment a little more comfortable. However, it is important to remember that all medications have side effects, and each situation should be evaluated independently to evaluate the benefit of the medication against its possible side effects. Remember, medications are not always

DSM-IV Criteria for Eating Disorders (cont.)

BINGE-EATING DISORDER

- Recurrent episodes of binge-eating. An episode of binge-eating is characterized by both of the following:
  - —Eating, in a discrete period of time (e.g., within any 2-hour period), an amount of food that is definitely larger than most people would eat during a similar period of time and under similar circumstances
  - —A sense of lack of control over eating during the episode (e.g., a feeling that one cannot stop eating or control what or how much one is eating)
- The binge-eating episodes are associated with three (or more) of the following:
  - —Eating much more rapidly than normal
  - —Eating until feeling uncomfortably full
  - —Eating large amounts of food when not feeling physically hungry
  - —Eating alone because of being embarrassed by how much one is eating
  - —Feeling disgusted with oneself, depressed, or very guilty after overeating
- Marked distress regarding binge-eating is present
- Binge-eating occurs, on average, at least 2 days a week for six months
- The binge-eating is not associated with the regular use of inappropriate compensatory behavior (i.e. purging, fasting, excessive exercise) and does not occur exclusively during the course of anorexia nervosa or bulimia nervosa.

DSM-IV Criteria for Eating Disorders (cont.)

EATING DISORDERS NOT OTHERWISE SPECIFIED

- For females, all of the criteria for anorexia nervosa are met except that the individual has regular menses.
- All of the criteria for anorexia nervosa are met except that, despite significant weight loss, the individual's current weight is in the normal range.
- All of the criteria for bulimia nervosa are met except that the binge-eating and inappropriate compensatory mechanisms occur at a frequency of less than twice a week or for a duration of less than 3 months.
- Associated with the regular use of inappropriate compensatory behavior by an individual of normal body weight after eating small amounts of food (e.g., self-induced vomiting after the consumption of two cookies).
- Repeatedly chewing and spitting out, but not swallowing, large amounts of food.

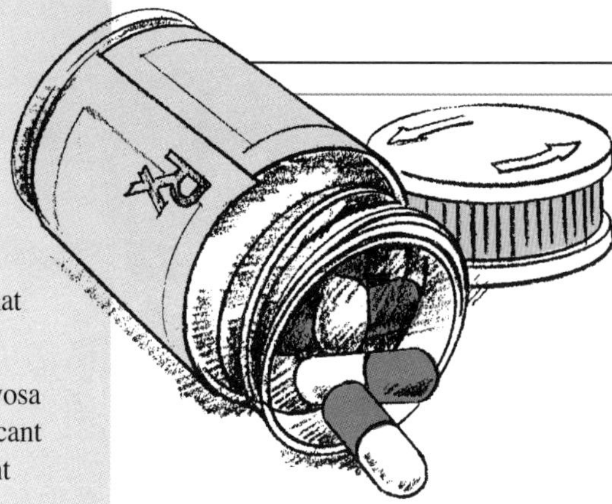

needed, and even when they are, not every medication affects each individual in the same way. In many cases, different trials of various medications may be required to find the one that works best for the individual.

Taking Your Medication

A Note for People with Eating Disorders

Many of the medications used in treating eating disorders require that you take them consistently for some time before you begin to feel the benefits. In particular, follow these guidelines:

- Take your medication specifically as directed. Many medications may have better effects if taken in the morning or at bedtime.
- It is important not to miss doses of medication as the level of the medication may fluctuate in the body and not reach a level where it can benefit you.
- Although some side effects with anti-depressant medications are common such as headache, nausea, or jitteriness, those effects will frequently diminish and go away if you continue taking the medication.
- Always report side effects to your health care provider as adjustments in the dose may be required.
- Studies show that long-term use of prescribed medications does not increase your risk for drug abuse.
- Your medication is prescribed only for you. Never share it with anyone.
- Do not mix alcohol with prescription medications. Skipping your medications on one day so you can drink alcohol does not work; medications remain in your system days after you take them.
- Do not stop medications abruptly. Withdrawl effects can occur, including headaches, nausea and dizziness.

The value in addressing the problem

Although eating disorders can take over people's lives, people can and do claim their lives back. The road to recovery begins when a person is able to "break the spell" of the eating disorder—to recognize the toll that the eating disorder is taking—physically, emotionally, socially, spiritually and then to make a decision to "turn against" the eating disorder and fight for his or her life. The journey is not easy and the challenges are great. Building a support team (family, friends and treatment professionals) is essential for standing up to the problem and beginning the recovery process.

CHAPTER 2

Common Myths of Eating Disorders

"People believe that you have to be bone thin to have an eating disorder."

–Jennifer, age 12

"People believe that when you go to the hospital you are all cured when you get out."

–Sam, age 16

"I thought that eating disorders just happened to teenagers. I didn't think that my eating behaviors could have long term consequences."

–Mary, age 41

Eating disorders have long been associated with numerous erroneous myths about the stereotypical patient and her or his family dynamics. A person who has an eating disorder is also likely to be very familiar with these myths. When asked what they perceive as the strongest eating disorder myths that prevail in society today, people with eating disorders have cited numerous examples, including the ones mentioned below. In one way or another, these assumptions can actually impair clients' recovery if they are not effectively dispelled and understood by family and professionals alike. Some of the common myths identified include the following:

Myth: Only women struggle with eating disorders.

This myth has unfortunately led to the misdiagnosis of men & boys struggling with eating disorders. In America, approximately one million males struggle with eating disorders, in part because of the increased emphasis in the media for men to achieve the "perfect" physique.

Myth: Eating disorders are about food. If the person struggling with the eating disorder would just eat, it would go away.

Our culture places such an emphasis on body size that it stands to reason that the individual finds himself or herself struggling with the issue of body size and thoughts of food. While in treatment, the client learns how to look at the underlying issues and not focus on the thoughts surrounding the size of their body. Recovery from an eating disorder involves repairing the damage that has been done to all aspects of a person's life. Eating normally is just one small part of the repair work.

Myth: Persons who have eating disorders are all slender.

Often, a person struggling with a binge-eating disorder or bulimia nervosa will have a normal physical appearance or may actually carry a bit more weight than they would if they were following a normal meal plan.

Myth: Everyone who is thin has an eating disorder.

This myth can be extremely frustrating for a person who has genetically inherited a more slender body type. If a person is truly struggling with an eating disorder, signs and symptoms—other than just a thin body size—will be present.

Myth: There is always something wrong in the family or the person with the eating disorder must come from a dysfunctional family.

This myth can be very painful for parents, especially mothers, who are often blamed for problems that their children experience. There is no proof that parents cause their children to develop eating disorders. Parents should be viewed as part of the solution—working alongside their children to help them break free from the problem.

Myth: Persons who develop eating disorders are weak-willed.

This myth actually tends to be the opposite of what is commonly seen in people with eating disorders. Typically, an individual with an eating disorder will be very strong-willed, competent, and high-achieving.

Myth: Recovering from an eating disorder is just like recovering from alcoholism.

Unfortunately in our society, many Americans struggle with alcoholism. It is common for a person struggling with an eating disorder to receive advice from someone recovering from alcoholism. Although such a conversation can be helpful in terms of sharing stories about tough struggles in life, the problem arises in receiving advice on how to recover. A person who recovers from alcoholism ultimately must stop drinking. They may stop going into establishments that serve alcohol and they may eliminate it from their home. A person struggling with an eating disorder cannot stop eating. Food must remain in the home, and "re-learning" how to eat in a healthy manner will be one of the many challenges.

Myth: When a person enters a treatment program, the problem goes away quickly.

This myth is difficult for everyone involved. The person struggling feels guilty if they cannot fix it quickly and the family becomes frustrated because they assumed treatment would make the eating disorder go away. Many say that the period of time following a hospitalization can be very difficult because people think they are "cured." Typically, however, they are just beginning the recovery process. Recovery may take one to five years, and for some individuals, it may be longer.

Myth: The only person needing support is the person diagnosed with the eating disorder.

This myth can again be problematic because often loved ones as well as other siblings need professional guidance. Assistance can be found by participating in family groups (with others who have a loved one struggling with an eating disorder), reading books about the topic, and seeking support from friends and relatives.

Myth: Eating disorders happen only to teens and people in their 20s.

Starvation diets and the cycle of bingeing and purging have long been considered afflictions of affluent white females in their teens and 20's. Although medical literature in recent years has shown eating disorders spreading across class, race and gender lines and striking girls at ever younger ages, the next large group of sufferers are middle-aged women. The anxieties of midlife - divorce, marital strains, parental deaths, empty-nest syndrome and menopause - are powerful catalysts for older women's eating disorders. Middle-age persons struggling with an eating disorder may be relapsing after overcoming eating disorders in their youth, or are experiencing them for the first time.

CHAPTER 3

Causes of Eating Disorders

Chains

O Little Girl in chains, what do you see?
A masquerade, red lips, a sparkling smile.

The discontented face stares back at me
And whispers, "I see monsters all the while."

O Little Girl in chains, you seem to frown
Can you see not your beauty where you are?

I only tell the truth. Please don't look down on me
On me. Oh, did you lose yourself? So far

You seem from Truth. I know you wish to fade
Away to nothing, growing thin by day.

Can you not see the damage you have made?
You call to me but then you turn away.

O Little Girl, your face is pasty white
And ghosts peer out your eyes which were once bright.

—Allison, age 15

One of the most commonly asked questions surrounding eating disorders is, "How did this happen?" As more adolescents and adults every year are exhibiting eating disorder behaviors, more families and friends are asking why.

While no single set of risk factors can be conclusively linked to eating disorders, we do have some hints as to how the process begins. Most are likely to be somewhere on a continuum of varying degrees of disordered eating behaviors. These behaviors will range from unhealthy eating practices (such as skipping meals and eliminating food groups from their diets) to diagnosable eating disorders. A practical way to outline the factors involved with the development of eating disorders is to chart them in this way:

sociocultural expectations of thinness

⇩

unhealthy body image

⇩

dysfunctional eating (disordered eating)

⇩

eating disorders: anorexia nervosa and bulimia nervosa and binge-eating disorder

Sociocultural expectations of thinness/unhealthy body image

Our society contributes tremendously to the development of eating disorders. The media perpetuates the ideal of thinness and the notion "the thinner you are, the happier you are." Cognitively, many of us can dismantle that message, although we have all fallen victim to it through unhealthy quick-fix dieting practices.

Dieting becomes a social phenomenon that affects many people in many adverse ways. They are bombarded with fat-free products, low-calorie foods, diet sodas, and overwhelmingly, the message "fat is bad." These messages often come to them inadvertently from people who are the closest to them: parents, teachers, coaches and friends. As individuals overhear conversations centered around the newest diet, weight loss and negative body image, the real message continues to be, "What a person physically looks like is more important than what's inside." When students learn about the negative effects of obesity and fat in health or nutrition classes, they often may miss the concept that dietary fat is necessary to one's health.

One of the last acceptable prejudices in the United States today is weightism. According to Michael Levine, PhD, an eating disorders expert, weightism refers to the prejudice that exists in our society today against people perceived as overweight. Individuals are extremely vulnerable to this message and very aware that being called "fat" is the worst teasing a person can be forced to endure.

Unhealthy body image is a byproduct of the sociocultural expectations of thinness. Throughout development, children tend to look to the media, their peers and their parents to determine what is expected of them. Often, the strongest influence comes from the media. As children become entrenched in the vastly unachievable images that the media projects, many children and adolescents develop an unhealthy body image. In

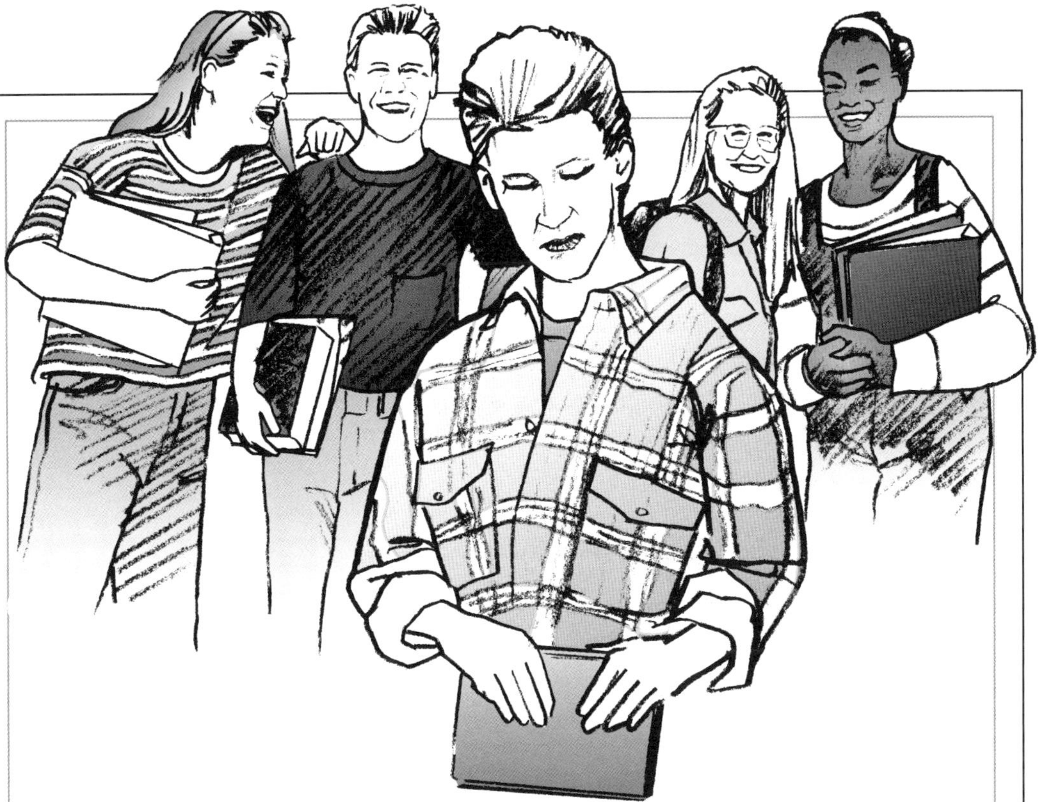

the process of feeling that they do not "measure up," they may also find that it is more acceptable to feel bad about their bodies rather than comfortable and good about them.

Both females and males are receiving mixed messages from the media. Although we are trying to teach children, "You are unique and should be an individual," they are hearing from the media that they should look exactly like one another. As a class of seventh graders described what girls and boys should look like, there was no consideration made for any variances from the "ideal" image, regardless of racial, ethnic or genetic differences.

> **Female:** "It is important to be thin and it leads to popularity and makes you have a good reputation. Body image is almost everything that matters."
>
> **Male:** "My image is to be fast with my hands and legs. It is also good to have a six-pack. It is good for your veins to stick out. The legs are the most important."

Because the first stage of the continuum is cultural expectations for thinness, it is important that parents, educators and students take a stand against unhealthy societal messages with anti-anorexia/anti-bulimia actions. An anti-eating disorder action may consist of eliminating fashion magazines and replacing them with magazines that focus on realistic images. Other anti-eating disorder messages would be placing higher importance on personal qualities such as being a good friend, caring about others, or being creative or determined. You may also want to strive to incorporate one-on-one time for discussion about this topic with your loved one.

Dysfunctional eating

The dieting industry grosses 40-50 billion dollars in the United States each year. In most cases, however, weight loss resulting from dieting—instead of healthy eating—does not last. The astounding fact about dieting is that between 98 to 99 percent of diets fail to produce permanent weight loss, meaning that most dieters will begin to put the weight back on after discontinuing the diet. Along with the weight gain comes a feeling of failure, low self-esteem, disappointment, and further pressure to find another quick-fix diet.

Normal eating versus dysfunctional eating

	Normal Eating	Dysfunctional Eating
Eating Pattern	Eating at regular times, having regular habits. Typically may be three meals a day and one or two snacks to satisfy hunger.	Irregular, chaotic eating; individual often overeats or undereats, skips meals, fasts, binges, diets. Or usual pattern is of eating much less or much more than the body wants or needs.
How eating is regulated	Eating is regulated mostly by internal signals of hunger, appetite and satiety. Individual usually eats when hungry, stops when full, is hungry at mealtime.	Eating often separated from normal controls of hunger, appetite and satiety. Often regulated by inappropriate controls such as "will power," a planned diet, calories or fat grams, emotional or sensory cues, sight or smell of food.
Function/purpose of eating	Eat for nourishment, health, energy. Also for pleasure and social reasons. Eating enhances feelings of well-being, makes one "feel good."	Eating often for reasons other than nourishment: to shape body, improve body image, seek comfort or pleasure, numb pain, relieve stress, anxiety, anger, loneliness or boredom. May feel uncomfortable after eating, and have feelings of guilt, shame or insatiable desire for more.
Prevalence	Infants, small children, persons who don't diet or interfere with normal eating. At this time, likely higher rates for males, lower for females.	Chaotic eating and undereating affect many girls and women in the U.S., perhaps at times as many as 50 to 80 percent age 11 and over who say they are trying to lose weight; also increasing numbers of boys and men. Consistent overeating may occur for both genders.

(For information, please see the section, "What is normal, healthy eating?" on page 38.)

SOURCE: Berg, Frances M. Afraid to Eat: Children and Teens in Weight Crisis. North Dakota: Healthy Weight Publishing Network, 1997.

Please note: The chart above is designed to provide a better understanding of the differences in eating behavior, the effects they can have on physical and mental functioning, and the value of normalizing eating behavior. It should not be used as a diagnostic tool, or to label children or adults.

Dysfunctional eating or disordered eating—the next stage in the continuum—typically occurs as a result of dieting. Eating "dysfunctionally" is not the same as having an eating disorder. However, the negative effects of dieting can be very similar to some of the symptoms that people with diagnosable eating disorders experience. It is important to understand what really happens when we diet—keeping in mind that not all diets lead to the development of an eating disorder:

- Tendency to binge eat. When we skip meals or drastically reduce calories, the brain and muscles continue to demand fuel. The increased demand causes rebound "munchies," usually for high-fat and high-sugar items.
- Inability to concentrate, being preoccupied.
- Potential for rapid weight gain. When we diet, we are eating far fewer calories than we should. As the body adjusts to getting less food, its metabolism lowers and fat is stored more easily from fewer calories.
- Obsessive thoughts about food and eating.
- A craving for more intense flavors such as sweet, salty and sour.
- Increased development of unhealthy body image. When dieting ends, weight is gained, which results in irritability and strong feelings of failure.
- Medical complications. People who are dieting may typically experience fatigue, lightheadedness or dizziness, apathy, constipation, sensitivity to cold or lack of energy.

Other risk factors

Typically, the development of an eating disorder is not merely from socio-cultural influences, although it is our society that allows so many people to connect a feeling of pride with weight loss. Again, as our media glamorizes thinness, one feels gratification as they meet the standards of thinness. For people who are on their way to possibly developing an eating disorder, comments regarding changes in their weight can serve as encouragement to continue dieting. Comments such as "I wish I had as much will power as you do" or "I wish I was as thin as you are" tend to glamorize the idea of weight loss.

In addition to sociocultural expectations of thinness, several risk factors may make a person more prone to the development of an eating disorder. These risk factors may include the following:

- adolescent developmental issues
- genetic predisposition
- psychological factors
- family issues

Taking action against teasing:

A message for adults

"I had been teased all my life about the size of my body. By the time I turned 14, I was so tired of the kids at school calling me fat, chubby and lazy that I decided there was just one way to make the teasing stop."

–John, age 14,
lost 50 percent of
total body weight

Teasing begins at a very early age and continues throughout adulthood. When immersed in the act of teasing and chiding, kids are very hard on each other. In fact, most adults can remember at least one stinging comment made to them during childhood and can still recall the hurt it caused.

Teasing is not a new phenomenon, but it is an act that can be prevented by not allowing it to prevail in our schools. Of course, teachers, parents and coaches cannot possibly monitor all behaviors, but they can impose consequences when they hear teasing taking place. They can also be good role models by not engaging in conversations that place a negative slant on body shape and size.

Risk factors are important to identify in young people because the more risk factors they exhibit, the more likely it is that an eating disorder may develop. Understanding these risk factors are critical to helping prevent eating disorders in adolescents and to support a loved one recovering from an eating disorder.

Adolescence

Adolescence is a time in which both girls and boys are at a very high risk for developing an eating disorder. This time in a person's life is both physically and emotionally challenging, as teens are changing on a daily basis. At this age, a person may be extremely comparative and will look to their peers, the media and the people they deem as role models for approval. Being unable to control these changes and yet wanting to look like everyone else, an adolescent may become frustrated and self-critical. Because the standards that the media portrays are so unrealistic, an adolescent may resort to dramatic measures to achieve his or her goals. During the teenage years, an individual may be striving for independence from parents; when a parent attempts to point out unhealthy behaviors of his or her child, conflicts may arise.

This time is also difficult specifically for teens who develop either late or early in comparison to their peers. A boy who develops late may struggle with self-image, believing he is "supposed" to begin to look and feel "masculine;" yet he may not if he sees himself as too short or too thin. A girl may struggle if she develops early, as she may not be emotionally ready for the response from others, especially any comments that may be sexual in nature. Likewise, if she is taller than others, she may perceive herself as "bigger" rather than "taller." Situations such as these are typical and often enhance poor self-image in teens.

Intimacy and dating also add to the body image issues. Peer pressure, as well as the media, may convince a teen that he or she is ready to experiment with intimacy. Individuals may find that in reality, they are not emotionally ready for such a situation. Intimacy specifically heightens issues of body image, as being touched prompts a person to focus more intently on his or her imperfections. Dating will also be emotionally difficult; again, teens may look to the media in order to assess what others deem as attractive. This reinforces the message to teens that physical appearance is extremely integral to one's identity and social acceptance.

Genetic predisposition

Studies involving twins have demonstrated that anorexia nervosa and bulimia nervosa have a hereditability factor of 50 to 80 percent. This means that some individuals have an inherited predisposition to develop an eating disorder. Genetic predisposition may help to explain why some adolescents who experiment with dieting may get "caught" by an eating disorder, while others do not. Although genetics appear to play an important role in setting the stage for an eating disorder to develop, it is important to acknowledge the significant role that Western culture plays.

Psychology/Personality

Some evidence suggests that certain personality traits increase an individual's risk to develop eating disorders. According to some research studies, two core predictors of anorexia nervosa are perfectionism and childhood anxiety disorders diagnosed by age 8.

In addition, individuals who have anorexia are often described as having similar personality traits, including a preference for routine and orderliness, difficulty adapting to change, a tendency to avoid risks, perfectionism and being emotionally reserved. Although these characteristics may be present before the eating disorder is diagnosed, these traits are usually accentuated by weight loss.

Family issues

Family dynamics are important to understand and are a key component in the recovery process. In situations of abuse (sexual, physical, emotional), alcohol/drug use, financial constraints and divorce/marital challenges, for example, it is important to address the issue and understand that individuals will look for a way to handle the stress. In a society in which we are focused on body weight and shape, it is common for an individual to attempt to gain control over the situation by controlling his or her physical appearance. It is important to emphasize that not every family affected by an eating disorder has issues described above.

CHAPTER 4

Eating Disorders and Physical Activity

For everyone, being involved in a sport can create social connectedness, confidence and fun. Unfortunately, being involved in a sport can also put a person at greater risk for developing an eating disorder. Persons participating in sports that require thinness or weight control can be at risk of developing disordered eating patterns. Examples of these types of sports are:

- Gymnastics
- Figure skating
- Wrestling
- Rowing
- Swimming and diving
- Cheerleading/dance line
- Distance running
- Ballet
- Jockeying
- Cross-country skiing
- Body building

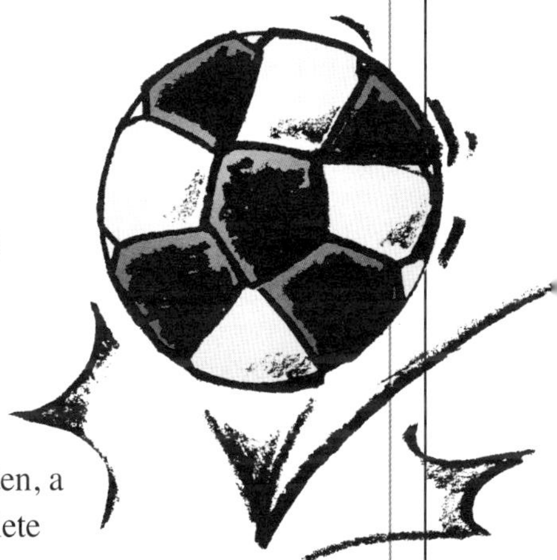

Athletes participating in these sports can be at risk by striving to achieve the ideal body for their chosen sport. Often, a message is being sent that "the leaner you are, the better athlete you will be." It is due to this message, in addition to the pressures that some people may be feeling, that they may begin to resort to unhealthy eating behaviors as a method of controlling their weight.

Another common situation that may arise for an individual is the dependency they may develop on exercise. One needs to think of food as fuel, rather than think of exercise as a mechanism to burn calories. Exercise is about building one's body, not erasing it. Often athletes develop different eating behaviors during their athletic season versus in the off-season. For some people, it is common for them to eat what they want during their season, but as soon as it is coming to an end, they begin restricting their caloric intake. They became dependent on the daily practices as a means to burn the calories they were consuming. Other athletes restrict more during their seasons. Typically, it is people involved in gymnastics, figure skating, ballet and cross country who do this as a way to perform better. Male wrestlers, who are often dual athletes (football players in

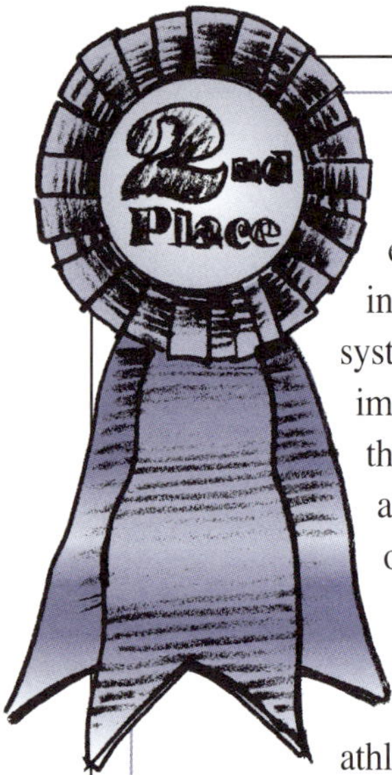

the fall and wrestling in the winter), bulk up during football and crash diet throughout their wrestling season. That type of behavior can be extremely harmful to the body. While a weight drop may initially increase speed, persistent lack of nutrition depletes the body's support system, resulting in decreased performance. Athletes need to be taught the importance of caloric and fat consumption during training, as well as throughout their off-seasons. Females need to be educated about calories and fat, especially because of their risk of developing amenorrhea and osteoporosis.

Educating athletes

Coaches play a significant role in the lives of their athletes. Young athletes turn to their coaches for both nutritional and athletic guidance. In fact, it is very common to hear a parent state, "My child will listen to her coach before she will listen to me."

For this reason, it is critical that coaches understand their role in their athletes' lives. An important part of that role is taking responsibility for conveying the appropriate nutritional messages to kids.

It is also important for coaches to remember that their athletes are individuals whose

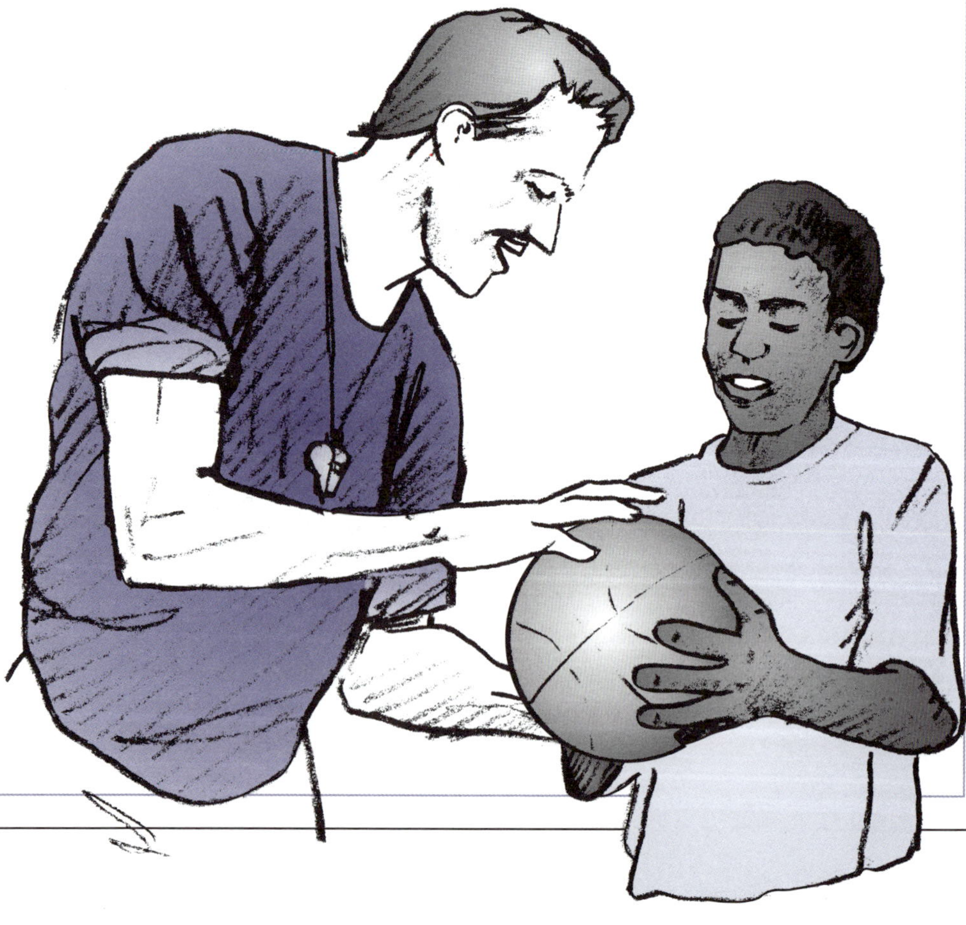

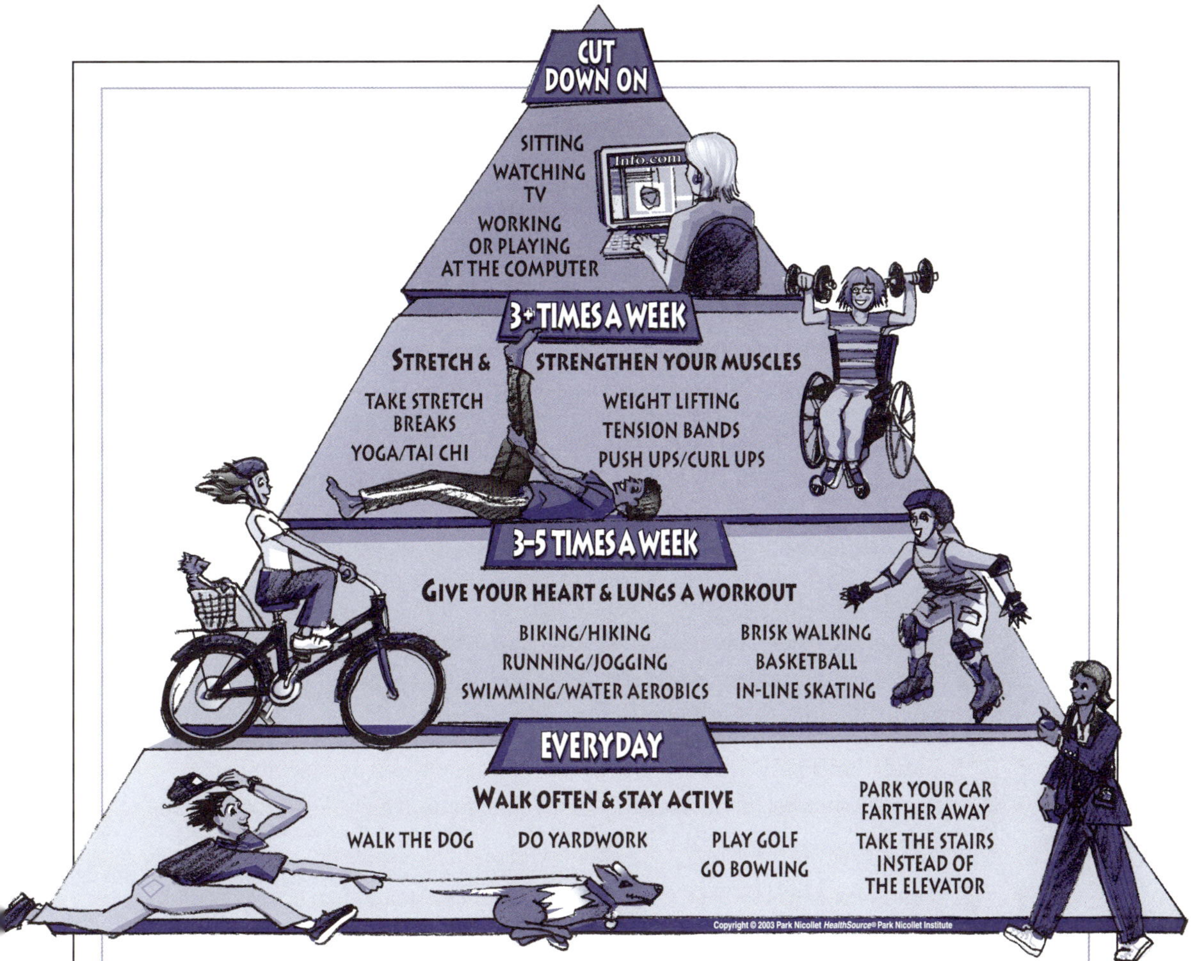

lives encompass many different activities and interests. Participation in sports is just a part of who they are. Many people who have battled an eating disorder have recounted that they felt that their whole identity consisted of being "a runner with the best time," "a center who was the best in the league." In some cases, this pressure of being the best in a chosen sport can be all-consuming and ultimately very damaging. Many coaches are playing a role in promoting balance in your athletes' lives by acknowledging the other aspects of their lives and by encouraging their athletes to have other interests. By focusing on the fun a person has in his or her sport, a coach can de-emphasize the competition felt among team members and eliminate the sense that they must sacrifice everything to "win."

Many tools are also available to assist you in sending out the right messages about food and activity. Registered dietitians also provide invaluable help; they can offer expert nutritional guidance during team meetings.

The Activity Pyramid, above, can help you send out the right messages about physical activity. It teaches moderation and helps reinforce the Surgeon General's message that physical activity need not be strenuous to be healthy.

You may choose to follow this model for "healthy exercise:"

H **stands for HAPPY**. First and foremost, healthy exercise should be fun and enjoyable.

E **stands for EATING.** You can't go far without the basics. Food is the basic energy source to fuel any exercise event. Fatigue takes the joy out of it.

A **stands for ACTION**. You need to move everything. Your exercise choices should include your arms, your legs, stomach—and yes, your brain. Move up, down, sideways, forward and backward—in any order! Cross training in between sports is great for keeping everything moving.

L **stands for LIFE**. Approach exercise as a lifetime adventure. You may rollerblade when you are 18 and waltz at 80, but the two are interdependent. Unrealistic short-term goals can cause physical and mental burnout—and leave little joy for the future.

T **stands for TIME.** Time is one of the top reasons why people do not succeed with healthy exercise. It takes time to do it right. Plan for it. Make it a priority. You are worth it.

H **stands for HARMONY**. Remember that magic word "balance." Listen to your body; if it hurts, your activity level is not healthy. Listen to your friends; if friends express concern about your exercise (by saying things such as "Hey, we never see you anymore"), consider their message.

Y **What are the WHYS behind your exercise choices?** Ask yourself, if exercise did not affect your weight, would you still do it? If your sole goal is weight loss, danger lurks ahead. You soon skip things such as warm-ups, stretching and cool downs, since they don't burn lots of calories. Certainly, weight can be affected by exercise, but weight loss shouldn't be the only goal. After all, what will happen once you lose the weight? Also, by building muscle, exercise can add weight. Broaden your goals, ask more from your exercise—pleasure, friendships, more energy. It has a lot to offer.

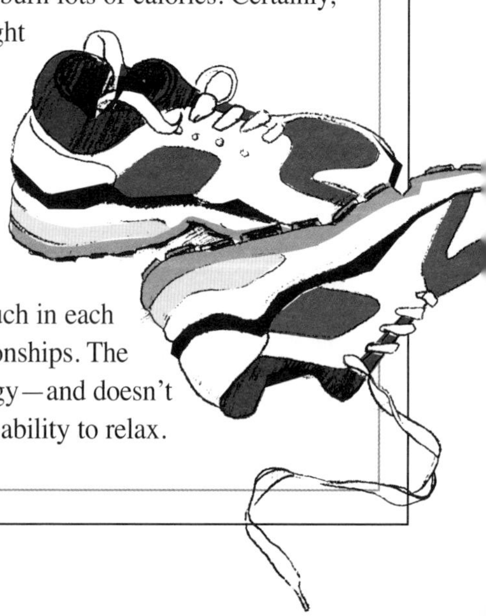

E **stands for ENERGY.** You only have so much in each day. You need it for work, school and relationships. The right exercise plan increases your total energy—and doesn't exhaust you. It improves your alertness and ability to relax.

X **stands for the little EXTRAS.** Sometimes, having fun with exercise just takes a little effort—correcting your foot placement, finding the right music or accepting that running in the rain means wet soggy feet. It also includes little pleasures such as a massage, a warm bath or plush new running socks.

E **stands for EMOTIONS.** Exercise is a mind trip, too. It should relieve your stress, not create it. It should include challenges and small risks that build your self-confidence, not overwhelm you. It should support time alone for thoughts and soul-searching. Other times, it is a key avenue for meeting others and fostering friendships. Teams can be a wonderful source for building relationships.

R **stands for ROLE MODEL.** Anyone who exercises is a role model for those around them, be it a friend or stranger. Healthy exercise acknowledges that responsibility and promotes the concepts presented in this list. Share your positive and negative experiences with others. Many appear to have the ideal body and brag about their physical skills, but they fail to mention that their school performance has declined and that their personal relationships are suffering from a lack of attention. Their days are consumed with food and exercise issues.

C **stands for CONSISTENT, not compulsive.** Have a plan, but allow flexibility. If a fever, finals or a friend in need conflicts with your exercise plan, remember the overall balance. Weigh the options, and consider moving the time that you exercise. On the other hand, if you have had conflicts every day this week, perhaps you need to stick to a plan. Take the time to think it through.

I **stands for INFORMATION.** Learn how to do your chosen activity properly. Read books, take lessons, talk with others, try new approaches. Does your activity support your goal? Are you doing leg lifts to eliminate fat on your thighs or build stronger muscles? Inaccurate information can lead to frustration and failure. Building friendships, sharing and expanding your mind are all part of that balance that exercise can offer.

S **stands for SUPPORT**. Support your friends, and let them support you. Offer encouragement, and take an interest in one another's goals. Applaud the effort, not just the outcome. Support your exercise with safety. Wear protective equipment, dress for the weather and learn the safety techniques of the sports you like.

E **stands for ENTHUSIASM.** Get excited. Enjoy your exercise. Keep trying new things. Look for indoor options, outdoor options, things to do alone, things to share, things to do when you mentally need a break, things to do when you need a challenge. Feed your spirit!

The signs of eating disorders in athletes

Knowing the signs and symptoms of anorexia and bulimia—particularly in athletes—is another important factor.

Anorexia nervosa, a serious life-threatening disorder characterized by deliberate self-starvation, is exhibited in athletes through the following signs and symptoms:

- refusal to maintain even a minimal normal weight consistent with the athlete's sport, age and height
- intense fear of becoming fat accompanied by repeated concerns by an athlete about being or feeling fat even when weight is below average
- periods of severe calorie restriction or repeated days of fasting or starving by eating only fruits and vegetables
- evidence of purposelessness, excessive physical activity (especially in a thin athlete) that is not part of the training regimen (e.g., extra sit-ups and laps)
- slowed heart rate and low blood pressure
- reduced body temperature and being sensitive to cold—cold hands and feet
- complaints of light-headedness and dizziness
- muscular weakness
- depression, irritability
- anti-social, isolative behavior
- perfectionism
- avoidance of water or excessive water intake

Bulimia is a serious life-threatening disorder characterized by recurrent episodes of binge-eating usually followed by self-induced vomiting or some form of purging as a means of controlling weight. An athlete who is suffering from this condition will have some of the following signs or symptoms:

- a pattern of eating substantial amounts of food followed promptly by trips to the bathroom
- consumption of huge amounts of food not consistent with the athlete's weight
- bloodshot eyes, especially after trips to the bathroom
- vomit or odor of vomit in the toilet, sink, shower or wastebasket
- wide fluctuations in weight over short time spans
- excess laxative use or evidence of use of diet pills or diuretics
- edema, particularly in feet and ankles, or hands
- tooth decay and gum disease
- headaches and fatigue
- perfectionistic: high performance and achievement expectations

- poor self-esteem coupled with shame and/or guilt
- depression
- a drive to exercise after eating

Addressing an athlete's eating disorder

Finally, it is important to know how to help an athlete who you suspect has an eating disorder. Here are some guidelines for reaching out:

1. The person who has the best rapport with the athlete should arrange a private meeting with him or her.
2. The tone of the meeting should be entirely supportive.
3. Calmly indicate to the athlete what specific observations were made that roused your concern. Allow the person time to respond.
4. Affirm and reaffirm that the athlete's role on the team will not be jeopardized by an admission that a problem exists.
5. If the information you receive suggests an eating disorder, share the following with the person:
   - You think the person has a problem with weight management, body image or both.
   - You are concerned about his or her health and well-being.
   - You are concerned that the matter needs to be evaluated by somebody who understands eating disorders.
   - Outside help is often required and this need should not be regarded as a failure or lack of effort.
6. Know about some of the resources in your school and your community (i.e., sports nutritionists, eating disorders programs) to which individuals can be referred.
7. Arrange for regularly scheduled follow-up meetings apart from practice times and obtain advice as to how you may continue to help. Participation on a team should be curtailed only if evidence shows that the eating disorder has compromised the athlete's health in a way that could lead to injury should participation be continued.

By being a positive role model, enforcing healthy eating and exercise habits, being aware of the signs of eating disorders, and knowing how to help, can have a positive impact on the lives of athletes—now and in the future.

CHAPTER 5

Modeling Normal, Healthy Eating Behavior

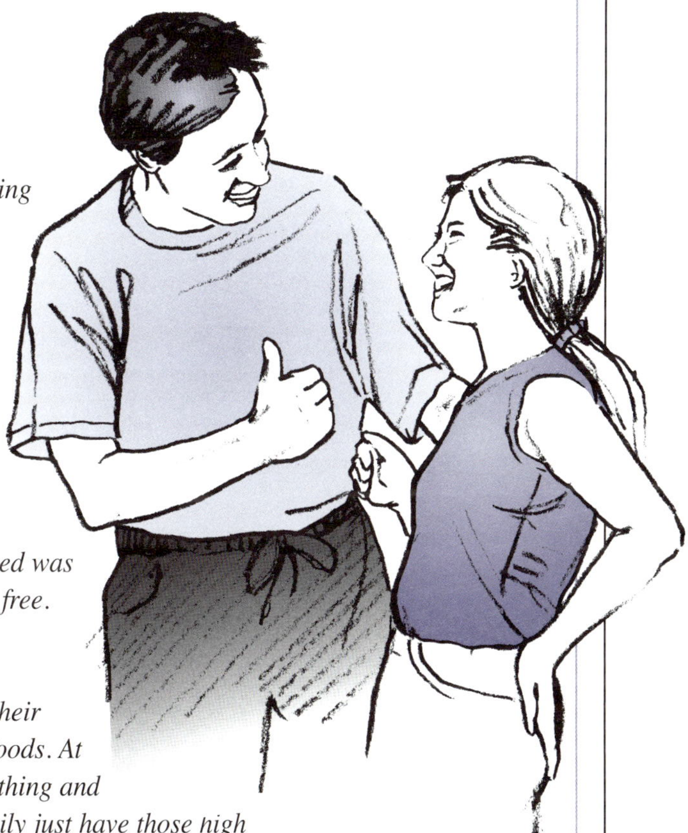

Kristen's Story

Kristen loved spending time and eating dinner at her friend Julie's house, even though dinnertime still made her feel anxious, there was something about dinner with Julie's family. They seemed to enjoy the food they ate! No one talked about the calories or fat content. No one was on a diet. They all ate normal amounts of food and had healthy weights. Another thing Kristen noticed was that none of the food was diet or fat free. They were just regular foods! This scared Kristen the most. She often wondered how the family stayed at their healthy weights while eating those foods. At her house they bought fat-free everything and were always dieting. Did Julie's family just have those high metabolisms people talk about, or was it more than that?

The philosophy that Julie's family holds about food and eating is becoming increasingly rare in America today. Often, Americans are so food- and weight-focused that the extreme efforts we put into achieving this "ideal" weight cause us to be preoccupied and even obsessed with our weight. (It is human nature to always want even more of what's being denied.) The same principle holds true for food. Therefore, we are often setting ourselves up for failure when we think about food and dieting.

Being a healthy role model

To be a healthy role model like Julie's family, ask yourself what type of message you are sending through your own eating habits and perceptions of body shapes. This self-analysis may include the following questions:

Eating habits

Are you buying primarily diet foods (including low fat and low carb) and beverages instead of regular foods?

Are you often skipping breakfast or other meals during the day or eating very low-calorie meals?

Are you skipping specific food groups such as milk/dairy or meat/protein to save calories?

Do you find yourself drinking large amounts of diet pop or water during the day instead of eating when you feel hungry?

Are you avoiding foods with fat?

Do you find yourself speaking in terms of food being "good" or "bad?"

Do you practice "black" and "white" behaviors such as (1) eating all or none of something or (2) never eating snacks or always snacking?

How much energy are you spending on issues related to weight and food (e.g., comparing body types or thinking about what to eat)?

Body shapes

Do you find yourself commenting on the weights and sizes of others?

Are you exercising solely to lose weight, and are you focusing on calories burned and pounds lost?

Do you feel guilty on days you don't exercise?

Do you wear uncomfortable clothes just because they make you look thinner?

Are you putting off things you've always wanted to do because of dissatisfaction with your body?

Do you avoid social situations because you are uncomfortable with your body? i.e., wearing bathing suits, etc.

Do you often think being thinner would make you happier?

If a day equals 100%, what percent of the day do you spend thinking about food, weight or body image?

Some of these questions may seem silly and others may make us think. Nonetheless, they are all important to consider if we want to help in the fight against eating disorders. Many of the people who are around you have a very good idea what your answers would be to most of these questions. It is always surprising how many messages we send to our loved ones (children, spouses, etc.) without even realizing it. Our nonverbal language and those ever-slight comments speak volumes.

Making changes

Making changes begins with assessing what your own attitudes and viewpoints are—and how you may be projecting these views on to others. Positive change occurs when we attempt to alter perceptions that may be negatively affecting ourselves and others.

Give pause to what "normal" means. Think about the direction society may be leading us. Too many have gone beyond what is "healthy" eating into an area where the quest for an "ideal" weight is of a higher priority than other areas of life. People come in many shapes and sizes. As individuals, we all have our own "healthy weight." It is one of the many things that makes us wonderfully unique. Thus, even if two people have the same commitment to healthy eating and physical activity, they are not likely to have the same body size and shape.

Understand the differences between healthy eating and dysfunctional eating (see pages 37–40). Know the characteristics of each so that you can educate others about their own eating habits and perceptions on weight.

Understand the difference between healthy physical activity and excessive or compulsive exercise. Healthy activity is pleasurable; it adds—not steals—energy. Ask yourself, "If exercise had no effect on my weight, would I still do it?" If the answer is yes, your activity is probably at a healthy level.

Take a look at some of the attitudes in other countries. Countries in Europe have very few commercially made diet and lowfat foods in their marketplace. They also do more moderate, consistent forms of exercise such as walking or biking to work and to the store. In Europe, food and dieting are less of a priority, and the attitudes of Julie's family are likely to be more common.

Examine your own viewpoints. As in other areas of life, before we can change others, or even have an impact on them, we need to address the negative attitudes we ourselves hold. Think about the type of views you are portraying to others—as a friend, teacher, coach, parent or spouse. If we don't change ourselves, we're of much less benefit in helping others.

Do your best to break our national obsession with physical appearance. Don't make comments or judgments about people's weight and appearance. Find inner qualities that deserve more attention.

Help people focus on enhancing their total health and well being—rather than losing weight or achieving a specific "ideal weight." Understand that an overall level of fitness is not dependent on the amount of fat on the body.

Realize that a certain amount of fat is needed every day. Dietary fat is a nutrient that helps the body transport and absorb fat-soluble vitamins such as vitamin A, D, E and K. It also helps the body make hormones and nerve cells and is essential for both the brain and eye retina.

Develop an understanding that improving a person's body image does not require changing one's actual body size, shape or weight. Improving a person's body image is a slow gradual process that can be achieved.

Refuse to let any insecurity you have about your appearance be an excuse that keeps you from doing the things you really want to do in life. Decide how you want to spend your energy: pursuing the perfect body or pursuing fun or enriching activities.

Identify situations that are best to avoid, such as reading certain fashion magazines, watching television shows that focus on body image or talking with friends who are continually dieting or talking about weight.

Promote mental, emotional, spiritual and physical nourishment in the following ways:

- Develop special gifts and talents.
- Wear flattering and comfortable clothes.
- Enjoy varied activities and expanded interests.
- Appreciate your abilities and attractiveness.
- Expand your friendships.
- Don't let the body or "shell" define who people are.

Learn to enjoy food. With such an emphasis on lowfat, high-fiber and weight-reducing fare, it can be difficult to truly savor what we eat without feeling guilty. Next time you eat, pay attention to the smell, texture and flavor of the food. Slow down and enjoy it.

Remember the function of your body parts, not just their appearance. Your legs allow you to walk; does the shape or look of them really affect their function?

Remember that society's definition of "beautiful" changes over time. Recognize how fleeting the present ideal really is.

What is normal, healthy eating?

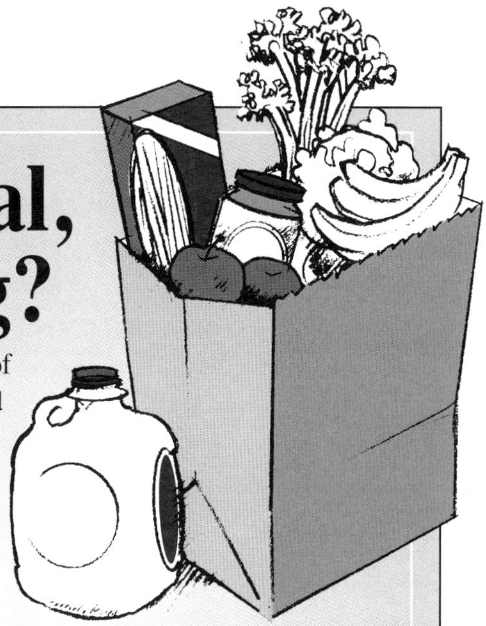

Many Americans have developed a distorted view of normal, healthy eating as a result of society's mixed messages. Americans are practicing a more restrained and chaotic type of eating with the goal of acheiving the ideal body weight and shape. As a result of such restrictive behaviors, normal eating can become dysfunctional eating and at times even escalate into an eating disorder.

Normal, healthy eating

Healthy eating usually means eating foods primarily for nourishment, health and energy but also for pleasure and social reasons. Internal signals of hunger, appetite and feelings of fullness regulate healthy eating. Healthy eating also promotes clear thinking, the ability to concentrate and mood stability.

Normal eating means eating foods from each of the following food groups – grains, fruits & vegetables, calcium-rich dairy foods, fats, proteins, and desserts. A healthy

The **Normal Eater's** Food Guide Pyramid

Eat mindfully.

Eat with others.

Include your favorite foods.

Choose a variety of foods.

Listen to hunger and satiety cues.

Eat at regular intervals.

balance of foods from all six food groups is needed to nourish and satisfy your body. The number of servings needed from each group to maintain good health varies for each individual and depends on factors such as current level of physical activity.

The Normal Eater's Food Guide Pyramid shows the importance of making a variety of food choices & the key behaviors that support normal eating. The shaded stripes on the pyramid represent various types of foods that are needed for good health. The Normal Eater's Food Guide Pyramid also shows that normal eating means focusing on key eating behaviors, such as how and when you eat, instead of just focusing on what you eat.

Benefits of Healthy Eating

Your level of functioning, both physically and mentally, depends to a large extent on the food that you eat. You need a balance of six nutrient groups (water, carbohydrates, protein, fat, vitamins, and minerals) in order to:

- think clearly and handle the mental challenges of everyday life
- stay alert
- look and feel your best
- promote physical strength and endurance

The key components of healthy eating include the following:

- eating normal portions
- eating in response to hunger and learning to stop when satisfied
- the equivalent of at least three non-dieting meals and snacks each day
- choosing diet foods or diet drinks in moderation
- avoid calorie counting
- eating some protein, fat, and carbohydrates at each meal

The following quote by author and dietitian Ellyn Satter is an excellent definition of normal eating:

> *"Normal eating is being able to eat when you are hungry and continue eating until you are satisfied. It is being able to choose food you like and eat it and truly get enough of it—not just stop eating because you think you should. Normal eating is being able to use some moderate constraint in your food selection to get the right food, but not being so restrictive that you miss out on pleasurable foods. Normal eating is giving yourself permission to eat sometimes because you are happy, sad or bored, or just because it feels good. Normal eating is three meals a day, most of the time, but it can also be choosing to munch along. It is leaving some cookies on the plate because you know you can have some again tomorrow, or it is eating more now because*

they taste so wonderful when they are fresh. Normal eating is overeating at times: feeling stuffed and uncomfortable. It is also undereating at times and wishing you had more. Normal eating is trusting your body to make up for your mistakes in eating. Normal eating takes up some of your time and attention, but keeps its place as only one important area of your life.

In short, normal eating is flexible. It varies in response to your emotions, your schedule, your hunger, and your proximity to food."

SOURCE: © Copyright by and reprinted with permission from *Secrets of Feeding a Healthy Family* by Ellyn Satter. Kelcy Press, Madison, WI 1999.

What stands out the most in this quote is the flexibility in normal eating. It's not perfect eating, but it's healthy eating. Humans aren't meant to be perfect.

Dysfunctional Eating

Dysfunctional eating is used to describe the abnormal, inappropriate eating that is becoming more common in the United States today. Dysfunctional eating is centered on eating for thinness, body shape and for comfort from stresses. Dysfunctional eating includes irregular or chaotic eating in addition to consistent undereating or consistent overeating.

A person with dysfunctional eating often feels tired or lacks energy, particularly if they are undernourished. An individual can often lose mental focus, alertness and the ability to concentrate on tasks. Often interest becomes narrowed and inward with a decrease in ambition.

Dysfunctional eating is rare for infants, small children, and others who have not dieted or interfered with the body's regular eating process.

Dysfunctional eating is affecting 50 to 80 percent of women and girls over age 11 and is increasing in boys and men.

Eating Disorders

When people struggle with an eating disorder, their thoughts often revolve around weight, food and calories. They may spend a significant portion of their day thinking about what to eat, how to burn off calories and how fat they are. They may also feel guilty for what they have eaten. The eating disorder mutes their ability to communicate with their bodies. People dealing with eating disorders are often unable to use body cues such as hunger or fullness to regulate eating.

Clues to an eating disorder:

A person who has an eating disorder may do the following:

- eliminate entire food groups
- skip meals and often say they're not hungry
- use lots of diet food, gum and water to feel full
- become isolated from friends and make excuses for not eating socially
- eat erratically—by overeating, undereating or eating fast
- constantly talk about food, calories and being fat—while eating erratically

If you know someone who exhibits any of these signs, he or she may have an eating disorder. For tips on getting help, please see Chapter Six: Getting Help (page 41).

Please remember: A person does not necessarily have to stop eating to develop anorexia. Many people today are eating and starving at the same time—by eating entirely only certain foods (such as fruits and vegetables) and eliminating essential nutrients (such as fat and protein).

CHAPTER 6

Getting Help

"My daughter just turned 12 years old and has suddenly decided that she will only eat one meal a day and is refusing to eat anything with fat in it. She's dropping weight and has gone from being a very cheerful adolescent to someone no one knows anymore."

—parent, sharing concerns during a phone screening

Because eating disorders can slowly sneak into someone's life, it is sometimes difficult to see the process evolving until an individual's personality, body weight or general appearance has changed dramatically. This can be a very frightening time for parents and loved ones, and addressing the situation can be very challenging.

Helping a loved one who may be struggling with an eating disorder can be difficult and confusing. Your role in the person's life can help you in how you approach the person and how the person responds to you. As a parent, sibling, friend, teacher or coach, you may have a special bond that will enable you to connect in a way that another may not.

An important thing to remember is that you are about to confront the person's greatest secret. The person may feel as though no one is aware of this secret or that someone may try to take it away. Be aware of the fact that the person you are talking with is going to feel a tremendous amount of fear related to their need to maintain this secret. You should be prepared for that fear—or, more commonly, the anger they'll have in response to wanting to cover up their fear. Anything that you can say or do to alleviate that fear will help to enable the receptiveness of your concerns for that person.

Getting it out in the open

When you talk to someone who may have an eating disorder, you will want to tell them of your concerns for them. Practicing assertive statements such as "I am worried about your health" or "I feel" can be useful in opening up the communication lines between yourself and that person. As you are discussing your concerns, you will want to state any changes you have noticed. This would include discussing personality changes as well as behaviors regarding food. For example, it can be beneficial for a person to hear

A note of caution:

There are certain signs that you need to look for when talking to a person who may be developing an eating disorder. If someone tells you that they are experiencing any of the following symptoms, make sure that he or she gets to an urgent care or primary care provider as soon as possible.

- ***bingeing and purging multiple times throughout the day***
- ***passing out***
- ***complaining of chest pains***
- ***complaining of severe stomach ache and/or vomiting blood***
- ***having suicidal thoughts***
- ***experiencing dehydration, rectal bleeding, anemia or impaired bowel functions—all of which can be related to the use of laxatives, diuretics or diet pills***

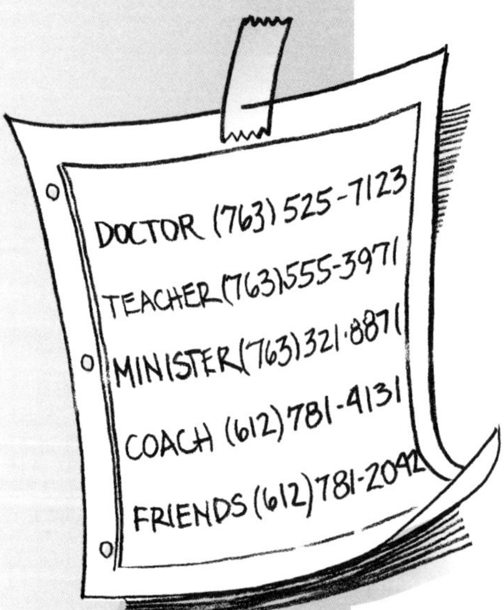

DOCTOR (763) 525-7123
TEACHER (763) 555-3971
MINISTER (763) 321-8871
COACH (612) 781-4131
FRIENDS (612) 781-2092

statements such as "I am concerned because last week at lunch I noticed that you did not swallow your food; instead, you spit it into a napkin that you later threw away." You may also want to note what effect the eating disorder is having on the person's favorite activities. These statements can have a powerful effect on a person with an eating disorder. For example, if a person loves basketball and his or her performance is lacking as a result of loss of energy, a coach may say, "You are a very talented basketball player and it frightens me that the eating disorder is stealing your energy from you." This comment can really ignite something within the person to fight against the eating disorder; the thought of losing the very thing that he or she feels most passionate about may be just enough to convince the person to seek help.

It is always a good idea to have resources available when you approach the person. Any written material that you can provide to the person may help identify the eating disorder within himself or herself. It is also a good idea to research available resources in your area. You will also want to locate facilities within your community that specialize in eating disorder treatment. Typically, your local hospital or clinic can offer you referral information to individual professionals in your area or treatment programs that specialize in eating disorders treatment.

Tips for family and friends

Jennifer's parents were at their wits' end. Jennifer had dropped weight and had become obsessed with having conversations about food, dieting, weight loss and how "fat" she felt. She no longer would join her family for dinner; she would make excuses such as eating at a friend's house earlier or needing to eat in her room so that she could finish her homework.

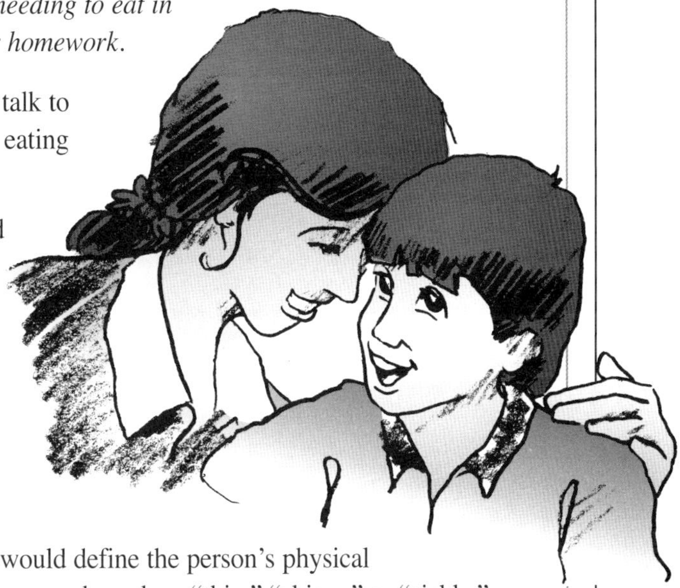

Following are some ideas on how to talk to someone who may be developing an eating disorder.

- Create a quiet, private and supportive environment for conversation.
- Share with the person the fact that you've noticed changes in him or her that concern you. Be specific.
- Don't use any words that would define the person's physical appearance. Stay away from words such as "thin," "skinny" or "sickly." Be aware that these terms define the exact body type that the person is starving to attain.
- Do discuss the changes in personality that you have seen in him or her (e.g., that he or she cries easily; rarely smiles anymore; or is crabby, edgy or withdrawn).
- Point out the things that you have noticed that they have already lost to a developing eating disorder—such as friendships, a bright smile, eagerness to participate in social activities, energy to participate in his or her favorite sports, or participating in events that involve food (pizza parties or birthday celebrations).
- Let the person share what he or she is thinking. Allow plenty of time for them to respond to your questions and concerns.
- Suggest that the next step be an appointment with the family physician, just to "check things out." If you are concerned about your child it is important to remind yourself that it is okay to be firm and that you are responsible for your child's well-being. (If symptoms of any other childhood illness were present, you would not hesitate to schedule an appointment with your health care provider.)

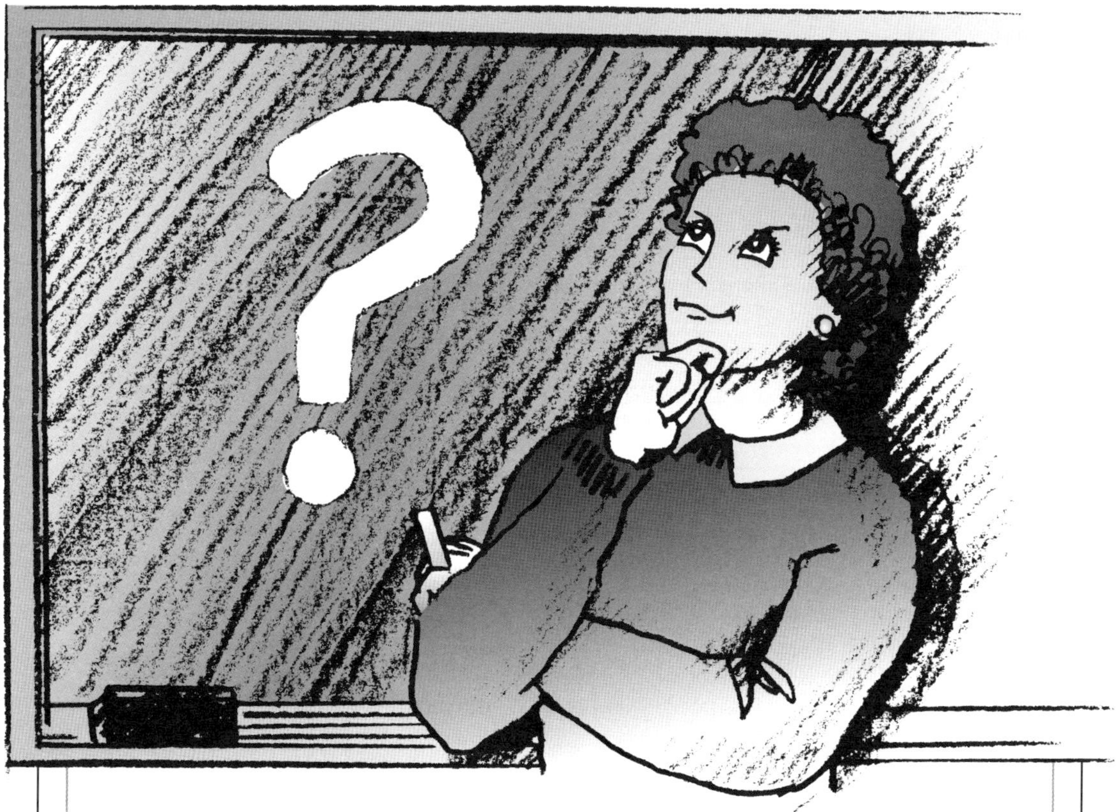

Tips for teachers and coaches

One day before swimming practice, three of Erin's friends approached their coach and asked to meet with her in private. Once in the coach's office, the three students told their coach that Erin had been throwing up after lunch every day for two months and that she had admitted to using laxatives. Erin's friends were scared for her and concerned that something would happen to her physically if she continued this behavior.

Following are some ideas on how a coach, teacher, school nurse or other supportive adult (in a school setting) can approach a student whom others suspect has an eating disorder:

- The adult who has the best rapport with the student should schedule a private meeting with him or her.
- Calmly share your concerns and let the student know that your main concern is his or her well-being.
- Establish a supportive tone to the conversation by reassuring the student that his or her "position on the team" or participation in school will not be jeopardized by admitting that a problem exists.
- Allow time for the student to respond.
- Reassure the student that the details of your conversation will remain

confidential. However, if necessary, you should be prepared to suggest a meeting with his or her parents to discuss making an appointment with a primary care physician.

- Always have written handouts on eating disorders available for the students and their parents.

A note on denial

In almost every case, denial will enter into the conversation. Fear or feelings of shame or guilt can trigger denial as well as a desire to hang on to the eating disorder. In some cases, the physiological effects that starvation has on the brain will prevent a person with an eating disorder from understanding why their loved ones are concerned. Thus, although it is very difficult to comprehend, a person who is starving continues to see himself or herself as "fat." He or she may live with the fear of being heavy and as a result will continue to deny that a problem exists. When the person denies that he or she has an eating disorder, concentrate on the person's emotional state, personality changes and what the person is losing as a result of the eating disorder.

Can I make it worse?

Remember that in some cases, the medical and emotional effects of an eating disorder can be irreversible and can cause the person years of pain and struggling. In severe cases, eating disorders can be life-threatening. For these reasons, you need to be reassured that you are doing the right thing by discussing your concerns with the person who you think may have an eating disorder. It is not unusual for the individual to be relieved that the issue is finally "out," and that he or she can now talk about what is happening.

Especially for students: How you can help

It can be very painful to watch a friend struggling with an eating disorder. Just thinking about discussing your concerns with your friend means that you are a very courageous person and terrific friend. The following tips can act as a guide for a friend reaching out to another:

- Speak to your friend privately after choosing a safe place to discuss your concerns. Your friend will appreciate feeling comfortable when he or she talks to you about such a difficult and emotional subject.

- Point out to your friend all of the things that you have observed that are causing you to worry.
- Let your friend know that you are concerned about his or her health and well-being and that you miss the person that was around before the eating disorder came into your friend's life. Point out changes in his or her personality and how this behavior may affect you (i.e., "I'm frightened by what's happening to you, and I don't like how you've changed.")
- Do not discuss with your friend your concerns about his or her weight or physical appearance. When you say, "You look so thin," your friend may interpret it as a compliment rather than a statement of concern.
- Allow your friend time to respond. Listening may be the best gift you can offer your friend. Remember that you may be the first person whom your friend has told, so he or she may really need to talk.
- Try to give your friend resources in your school and community (school nurse, school counselor, eating disorders programs, web sites on eating disorders). Offer to go with your friend when he or she talks to an adult.
- Your friend will probably ask you to keep this a secret. Don't tell other friends, but encourage your friend to confide in an adult. Talking to an adult is important; eating disorders can be very harmful, and your friend may need help.
- Be sure to listen for the following medical complications that your friend may say he or she is experiencing. If any of these complications are occurring, notify an adult immediately. Do not wait for your friend's permission.

  -bingeing and purging several times each day

  -passing out or having severe chest, stomach or back pains

  -vomiting blood

  -discussion of suicide

Remember, eating disorders are very serious and can be life-threatening. It is extremely important that you talk to an adult about what your friend has told you. It will also be a good idea for you to talk to a school counselor or adult with whom you feel comfortable; you may be overwhelmed with feelings regarding your friend's struggle. Remember that confronting your friend takes a lot of courage. Many people hope to have a friend as caring as you are.

CHAPTER 7

Treating Eating Disorders

Eating disorders are treatable problems. Throughout the past 25 years, significant advancements have been made in understanding and treating anorexia nervosa and bulimia nervosa. Treatment often takes many years, and a person's journey to claim his or her life back from these problems often involves a winding path with many detours. The important thing to remember is that recovery is possible.

Eating disorders exact a huge toll—physically, emotionally, socially and spiritually—on the lives of people struggling with these problems. It also affects family members and friends. A father who supported his daughter through the recovery process once likened the experience of eating disorders treatment to running a marathon when you expected only to run a sprint.

This chapter provides information about treatment and the process of recovery from eating disorders. If someone you know has been diagnosed with an eating disorder, this chapter will provide you with information that will help you support him or her.

What to expect

Before selecting a treatment program, it is important to understand the process for enrolling in a program. Many programs follow the process outlined below.

Telephone screen

Before a person enrolls in a particular program, a brief screening interview may be conducted over the phone. The purpose of this phone screen is to determine the following:

- If the person could benefit from a comprehensive eating disorders assessment.
- If the situation is urgent and the person should be medically assessed as soon as possible.

Direct Admissions

A patient may be admitted directly into the inpatient, partial hospital or residential treatment programs. Direct admissions require referrals from primary care physicians, psychiatrists, other eating disorder programs and hospitals. Data regarding the patient's present physical and emotional status will be requested from the referral source and evaluated by the treatment team to determine appropriateness of a direct admission. The data also helps treatment specialists determine which treatment program is best for the patient.

Initial Assessment

If the information gathered during the intial phone call does not indicate that the person's situation warrants urgent attention, then an initial assessment will most likely be recommended. A comprehensive, assessment will take several hours and will help determine at which point the patient enters the treatment program. An assessment will typically consist of:

- a physical and medical examination, including lab work and an electrocardiogram (EKG)
- a nutritional evaluation
- psychological and psychiatric consultations

In care centers that provide comprehensive services, typically a care coordinator will be designated at the time of the initial assessment. This care coordinator will monitor the patient's progress through each phase of the treatment process and will coordinate the treatment plan with the patient and family, team members and insurance companies.

Selecting a treatment program

Often, seeking a referral from a friend, relative, teacher or physician is the best way to initially select a program. (A parent of a child who has gone through treatment can be an excellent resource when looking for an eating disorders program.) During the process of researching treatment centers, it is important to look for the following components:

A multi-disciplinary team approach

Helping a person to break free from an eating disorder usually requires a multi-disciplinary team of professionals with training in medicine and psychiatry, nutrition, exercise physiology, psychology and family therapy—and who have experience treating eating disorders. Keep in mind that eating disorders are very complex and require the expertise from many different professional clinicians; it is important to be wary of a sole practitioner who offers treatment for eating disorders.

Tips for seeking treatment:

- Inquire if the following disciplines are represented on the team: medical doctor, psychiatrist, registered dietitian, and licensed psychologist.
- Make certain that all of the care providers are licensed.

Treatment options

Every person struggling with an eating disorder should be able to access the appropriate level of care that they need to defeat the problem. There are different primary types of care that people can receive when they are diagnosed with an eating disorder.

Inpatient treatment. Treatment in a hospital will be recommended for persons requiring 24-hour medical monitoring because of medical problems caused by starvation and other eating disorder symptoms such as electrolyte imbalances, EKG abnormalities or severe depression/suicidal thinking.

Partial hospital treatment. This is a program designed to provide support, education, nutritional and medical monitoring and accountability during the hours of the day most identified as troublesome for patients struggling with an eating disorder. These clients participate in structured meals and therapeutic groups and activities during the day and go home at night.

Intensive Outpatient treatment. Intensive outpatient program is held several hours per day, twice a week and includes group and individual therapy. Skills learned in the partial and inpatient programs are practiced, as clients build confidence in their ability to change behaviors.

Outpatient treatment. The majority of patients with eating disorders are treated on an outpatient basis, where they come in one to three times per week. Outpatient treatment usually involves meetings or consultations with the following:

- a dietitian—for assistance with meal plan compliance
- a physician—to monitor medical status
- a psychiatrist—for medication management
- a psychologist—for psychotherapy (group, individual and family work)

Residential care. A small number of individuals whose lives have been taken over by these problems for many years may need the support of a longer-term residential treatment program to help reclaim their lives. This program offers longer therapeutic support (up to six months) in a less acute environment.

A note on insurance coverage

Because treatment can be costly, we suggest you call your insurance company and verify your mental health benefits. The toll-free customer service number can be found on your insurance card. This can be a very emotional and stressful time, so it is recommended that the financial details be investigated before the first appointment.

A collaborative treatment approach

To defeat anorexia, bulimia, or binge-eating disorder, cooperation and mutual respect is imperative—among the treatment team, the person with the eating disorder and his or her family and friends. People diagnosed with anorexia or bulimia should never be referred to as "anorexics" or "bulimics;" they are people, not "ics." Their strengths and problem-solving abilities—and their families' support—should be an active component of treatment. Acknowledging the significant role that society plays in the development of eating disorders is also an important part of the collaboration. Recognizing the role of these external influences allows the person and their family to fight against the problem, rather than against themselves or one another. People who have broken free from eating disorders can also play an important role in the treatment, offering hope and inspiration through their stories.

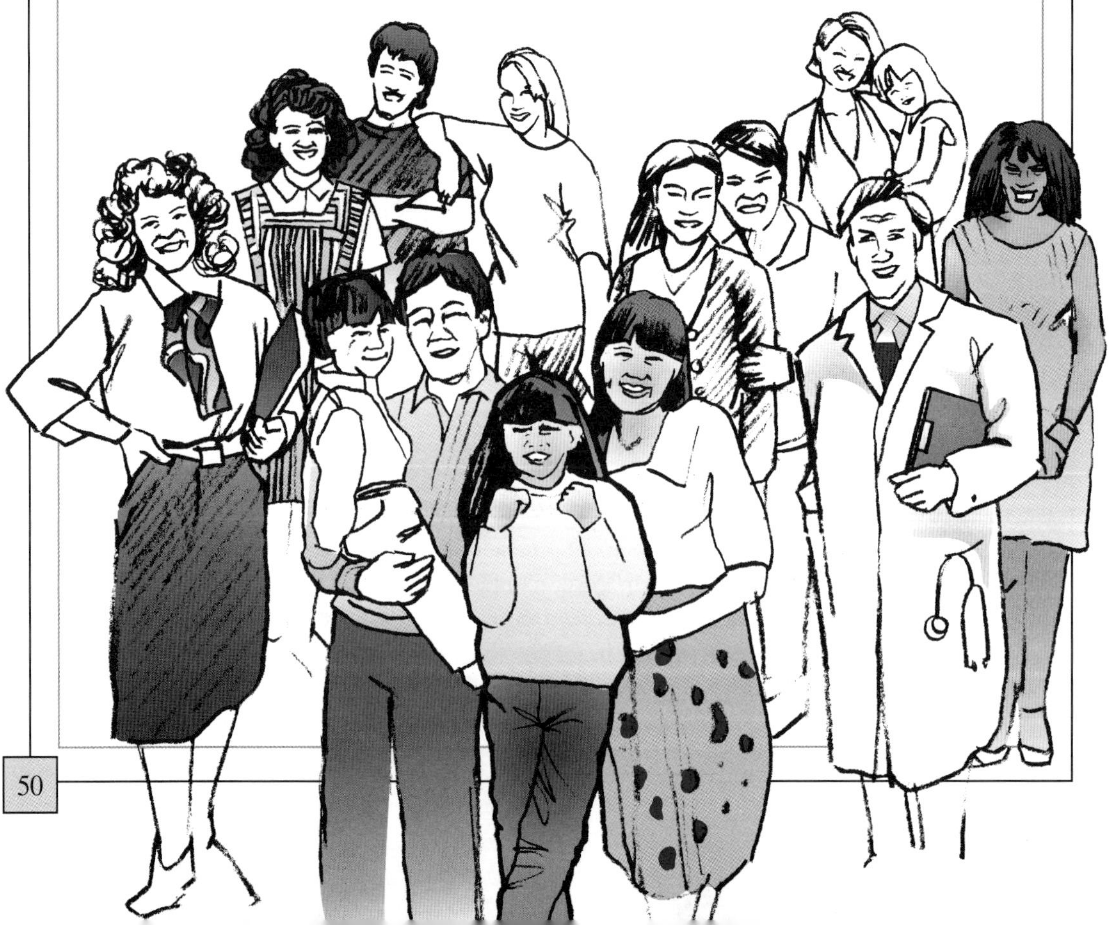

The outcome

Ultimately, with treatment, about 60 percent of people with eating disorders recover. For those who overcome eating disorders, it usually takes a long time, perhaps an average of five-seven years of slow progress that includes starts, stops, slides backwards but also significant progress. With patience and support, people with eating disorders can and do move steadfastly toward better mental and physical health.

Breaking Free from Anorexia/Bulimia:

One Person's Journey Through Treatment

Brittany,[1] age 13, did not have a choice about being hospitalized. Her physical condition necessitated inpatient treatment. She was admitted with abnormal heart rhythms, severe dehydration and significant weight loss. Depression also had Brittany in its grip.

During the initial visits, the care team learned that Brittany had lost her grandfather the previous year. Her grandfather had been her biggest fan at all of her figure skating events. Now he was gone. Brittany kept skating because she wanted to excel for him.

Her body started changing as she moved into adolescence. She needed to remain petite and light to execute the jumps and lifts that would make her a winner. She began cutting back on food. She started a pattern of not eating unless she exercised. She began avoiding her friends so she could exercise. Anorexia/bulimia took over.

Brittany began her nine-month journey to claim her life back from anorexia/bulimia in the hospital. The first step of that journey was to reclaim her physical health. Brittany needed to eat again.

Initially, Brittany ate all of her meals and snacks in the inpatient dining room with her peers on the unit. She was expected to eat all of the food that was selected by the dietitian or to drink a liquid replacement for food not eaten. Although eating again after months of semi-starvation was very hard, Brittany acknowledged that it was a relief to not have to make a decision about whether she was going to eat and what she was going to eat at each meal. Brittany made it very clear, however, that it was peer support that got her through those first meals in the dining room. Anorexia/bulimia relentlessly stalked Brittany before she went into the dining room—

(continued on page 58)

telling her that she was going to get fat. And anorexia/bulimia followed her out of the dining room—ordering her to go into her bedroom and secretly exercise to burn off calories. But while she was eating, the camaraderie that she established with the women at the dining room table silenced anorexia's voice. It was a remarkable accomplishment.

Brittany said that it made a huge difference that everyone else was eating and that some people who had been in the program longer were eating even more food than she was. Peers confirmed from their own experience what the medical team had told her—that the bloating and discomfort that comes from refeeding eventually goes away. And she came to believe that this was true. Her friends on the unit—and they clearly did become her friends—cheered her on when she ate a hamburger for the first time in 18 months.

The dietitian worked closely with Brittany to help her to feel as much in control of the refeeding process as possible. After the first few days, Brittany began to take a more active role in food choices. When her meal plan was increased, she would work with the dietitian to add foods to the plan that she believed she could manage to eat. The dietitian gently but firmly challenged her to increase the variety of foods that were "safe" to eat. Brittany constructed a list of foods she had enjoyed eating in the past but that anorexia/bulimia had stolen away from her. Pizza was at the top of the list. Gradually Brittany began checking these foods off—like the hamburgers—when she claimed them back.

Eventually Brittany graduated to "meal group" and began reclaiming her control in both cafeteria and restaurant settings, selecting foods from a wide variety and returning to eating in public. To help her to transition back to home, she planned a family meal to become reacquainted with what it was like to eat with her family. Meals at home before the admission had been stressful and painful, with her family feeling like the food police. Everyone wanted this to be different when Brittany returned home.

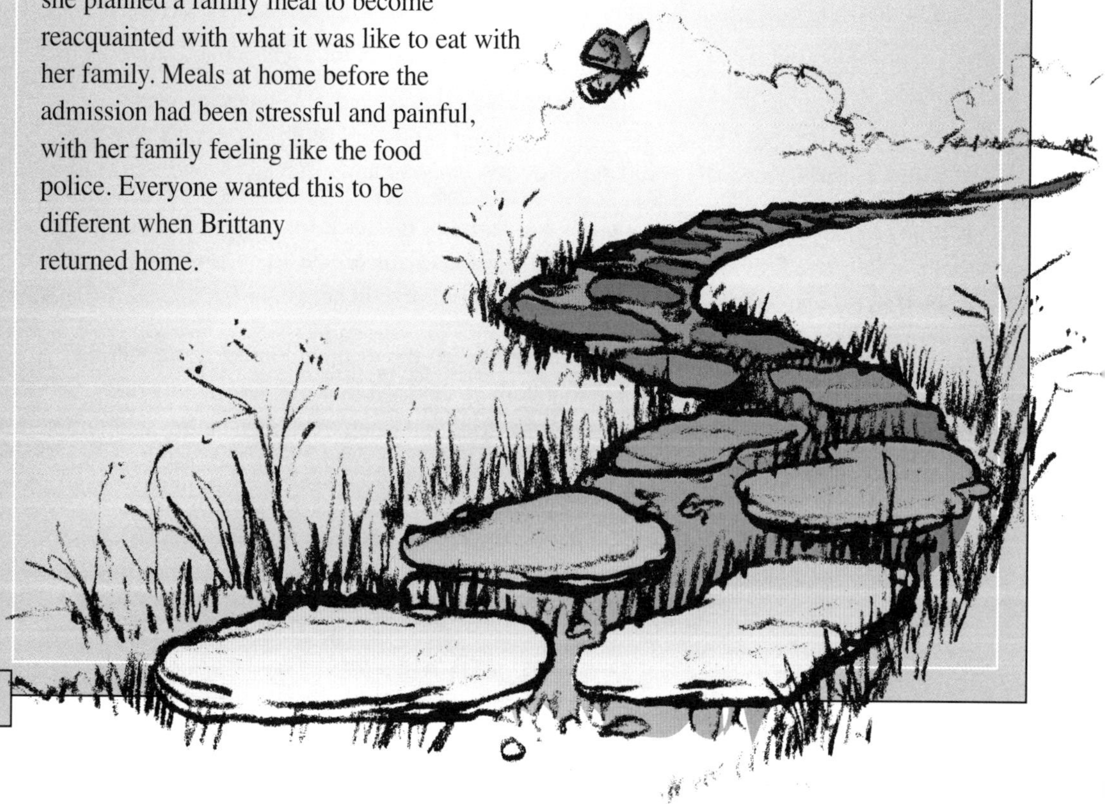

Reclaiming her physical health in order to skate again became a strong motivator for Brittany to beat anorexia/bulimia. While in the hospital, however, her body was weeks away from being strong enough to skate, even for 15 minutes. Brittany was able to participate in a stretch group, led by the physical therapist, where she learned to reconnect with her physical self in a gentle way. In addition to experiencing the sheer joy of movement, Brittany worked on flexibility and coordination.

She even tried both hands at non-perfectionistic juggling. As her physical health improved, she began strengthening exercises—weightlifting. But her heart rate remained too low to participate in any aerobic activity before she was discharged.

During her treatment, she also attended occupational therapy groups. It was here that she began to give physical form to her experience with anorexia/bulimia. She drew an image of herself driving into a tunnel with anorexia/bulimia in the passenger seat. When her car emerged from the tunnel, she was in the passenger seat with anorexia/bulimia at the wheel. This allowed her to explain how subtly she had been "captured" by anorexia/bulimia. She also discovered similarities with others as she created a list of "promises" that anorexia/bulimia had made to her, including: "you will be more popular," "guys will like you better," "you will be a stronger athlete," "you won't be lonely," "people will respect you" and "you will be in control." Together, they recognized that the promises made by the eating disorder were false. Brittany decided to install an ejection seat in the passenger side of the car!

The psychiatrist prescribed an anti-depressant to help her to stand up against depression. This medicine also helped to mute anorexia's relentless badgering about weight, food and calories. Brittany also took a medicine to help her to digest food.

Initially, psychotherapy focused on supporting Brittany to choose whether or not to smile. She carried a lot of sadness about her grandpa but always wore a smile. She began to take the risk of showing her sadness to others. She began to talk about her grandpa. She also began to talk about how isolated and alone she felt, wondering if she would ever fit in with friends at school.

Brittany and her family began to look at the ways that anorexia had taken over the lives of everyone in the family. Brittany's mom was able to talk about her feelings of being responsible for causing the eating disorder—"if only she had been a better mother." Brittany's dad talked about his frustration with not being able to "fix" this problem that his daughter was struggling with—"fixing problems is a dad's role." Brittany's sister was able to share that she was mad that her sister was getting so much attention and scared that Brittany was going to die. These honest conversations helped family members to join together to fight the problem—anorexia—rather than blame themselves or each other.

Brittany also took the risk of inviting two friends from school to attend multi-family support group with her parents and sister. This group—filled with people struggling, both family and friends—helped her friends to learn about eating disorders and how to support Brittany in her recovery. It was clear that Brittany was building an unstoppable support team.

As Brittany was approaching discharge from the hospital, she, her parents and team members met together for a care conference. At this meeting, they all celebrated the steps that Brittany had taken to claim her life back from anorexia and bulimia. They also discussed the challenges that lay ahead. There was unanimous agreement that transitioning to partial treatment was the best anti-anorexia/bulimia strategy that Brittany could make.

Partial treatment, Brittany learned, was similar to inpatient treatment but only seven hours each day. She ate lunch and dinner with peers but had breakfast at home. She also got to sleep in her own bed at night. She attended therapeutic group activities and continued with individual and family therapies.

It was during partial treatment that Brittany took more time in therapy sessions to talk about her grandfather and her sadness about losing him. She also celebrated their close bond and her happy memories.

Her life was beginning to have more balance to it—school and homework, time with family, time with friends, time for skating. Brittany was ready for the next step: outpatient follow-up.

In outpatient follow-up, Brittany continued in individual and family sessions. She also joined an adolescent outpatient group. Some of the people who had been in the hospital were in this group. She saw the doctor and dietitian one time per week for medical follow-up. As her medical condition continued to improve, frequency of visits decreased. When stressors came up—difficulties with friends at school in particular—depression would rear its ugly head. Anorexia/bulimia's voice would return more strongly at these times, too. She and her mom and dad rode through these times, and they became less problematic. As treatment was winding down, frequency of visits decreased to one time per month.

Near the end of her treatment, Brittany surprised her friends, family and care team all by informing them that she was planning to stop figure skating competition. She announced that she was joining the girl's hockey team at her school. Many of her friends were making the switch from figure skating to hockey because, as Brittany put it, "With figure skating there is so much pressure to perform, to be perfect; with hockey you just go out there and have fun."

[1]Some details of Brittany's story have been changed to protect confidentiality. We would like to thank Brittany for allowing us to share parts of her experience of claiming her life back from anorexia/bulimia.

CHAPTER 8

Seeking Additional Help

You may have a friend or loved one who is exhibiting signs of an eating disorder and you're wondering how to help him or her get the treatment they need. If you are like most parents who have a child diagnosed with an eating disorder, you probably have had moments of loneliness. You have probably experienced feelings of frustration, guilt, anger, fear and thoughts of where to turn next. You may be a teacher witnessing the culture changing from when you were in school and have noticed the attention paid to body weight and shape. You have probably felt frustrated and confused about what your role can be. You are not alone. There are many organizations, treatment centers and resources that can help you cope with your child's or friend's eating disorder issues surrounding body image, food and dieting. Here are a few suggestions.

The Primary Health Care Provider

If you can identify signs and symptoms of eating disorders in your loved one, the primary care physician should be contacted. Some insurance companies require that you see your primary caregiver first, then a specialist. Typically your primary caregiver will have knowledge on the topic and can assist you in the area of identifying any medical complications as a result of an eating disorder.

Specialists

There are numerous eating disorder programs throughout the country. Discuss with your primary caregiver what specialists are available in your area, including therapists, dietitians/nutritionists, physical therapists or exercise physiologists. In addition, most schools will have a counselor available on staff who will be knowledgeable in this area.

What you can expect, what you can do.

A person who has been or is being treated for an eating disorder needs support and encouragement to work toward recovery. In addition to providing that support, it helps to understand what the person is experiencing on the road to recovery—and what can aid or hinder their healing process. Their family and friends will also need encouragement and support.

People who are being treated or have been treated for an eating disorder…

- ***will have a "meal plan." Diet foods are not a part of the recovery meal plan (except an occasional diet soda).***
- ***are expected to have a schedule for regular meals and snacks.***
- ***may miss some school or work to attend eating disorder support groups or go to medical appointments.***
- ***don't want comments about how they look, their weight, how much they have gained or what they are eating.***
- ***will have an exercise plan with limits and progressions.***

Eating Disorders Resources

Academy for Eating Disorders, www.aedweb.org

Anna Westin Foundation, www.annawestinfoundation.org

ANRED: Anorexia Nervosa and Related Eating Disorders, www.anred.com

Dads & Daughters, www.dadsanddaughters.org

Eating Disorder Referral and Information Center, www.edreferral.com

Eating Disorders Coalition, www.eatingdisorderscoalition.org

Ellyn Satter Institute, www.ellynsatter.com

Gurze, Eating Disorders Resource Catalogue, www.bulimia.com

Media advocacy organization, www.about-face.org

Methodist Hospital Eating Disorders Institute, St. Louis Park, MN 952-993-6200, www.parknicollet.com/EDI

National Eating Disorders Association, www.nationaleatingdisorders.org

Recommended Reading

Berg, Frances M. ***Children and Teens Afraid to Eat: Helping Youth in Today's Weight-Obsessed World.*** Hettinger, ND: Healthy Weight Network, 2001.

Berg, Frances M. ***Women Afraid to Eat: Breaking Free in Today's Weight-Obsessed World.*** Hettinger, ND: Healthy Weight Network, 2001.

Freedman, PhD, Rita. ***Body Love: Learning to Like Our Looks and Ourselves.*** Calsbad, CA: Gurze Books, 2002.

Friedman, Sandra Susan. ***When Girls Feel Fat: Helping Girls Through Adolescence.*** Firefly Books, 2000.

Johnston, PhD, Anita. ***Eating by the Light of the Moon.*** Carlsbad, CA: Gurze Books, 2000.

Methodist Hospital Eating Disorders Institute. ***Journeys – True Stories of hope and recovery from those who have lived through an eating disorder,*** 2004. Call Park Nicollet Stores toll free 1-800-862-7412 x2662. www.parknicollet.com/stores

Methodist Hospital Eating Disorders Institute. ***The Journey Toward Freedom – Rediscovering the Pleasure of Normal Eating,*** 2006. Call Park Nicollet Stores toll free 1-800-862-7412 x2662. www.parknicollet.com/stores

Satter, Ellyn. ***Secrets of Feeding a Healthy Family.*** Kelcy Press, 1999. www.ellynsatter.com

Schaefer, Jenni. ***Life Without Ed.*** New York, NY: McGraw-Hill, 2004.

Here are some things that you can do for someone who is recovering from an eating disorder:

- ***Devote a few minutes each day to check in with the person. Ask the person to specify what would be supportive rather than "policing."***
- ***Understand the person's meal plan by attending nutritional consultations with his or her dietitian.***
- ***Make home an "eating disorder-free zone" by getting rid of all diet foods.***
- ***Offer to work together on menu planning and grocery shopping.***
- ***Keep the eating disorder out of the kitchen.***
- ***Give praise for hard work.***
- ***Spend the majority of conversation time on the aspects of the person not related to the eating disorder.***
- ***Have meals and snacks with the person. Having regular family meals is very important to the recovery process.***
- ***Avoid comments about the person's weight or appearance.***
- ***Exercise with the person.***

This book was developed by Methodist Hospital Eating Disorders Institute in Minneapolis, Minnesota. Funding support was generously provided by Park Nicollet Foundation.

Authors/Contributors

Carol T. Tappen, BA
Sadie Norby Gardner, BA
Joel P. Jahraus, MD
DuRanda Rinden, RD
Lois Neaton, PT
Irene Bugge, PhD
Elke Eckert, MD
Lianne Beyerl, OTR
Betsy Christopherson, MS, RD, LD
Kirsten Larsen, OTR
Jeanne Mettner
Cindy Schallock, BA
Kate Butitta, MPH, RD, LD
Jill Gorius, MD
Julie Lesser, MD
Shannon Simper, MBA
DeeAnn Swanson-Gritti, RN

Reviewers

Lyn Schroeder
Kay Leflay
Bob Knutson
Aimee Schaefer
Joel P. Jahraus, MD
Irene Bugge, PhD
DeeAnn Wozniak, RN, BS
Jane A. Norstrom, MA
Julie Mowery, RD
DuRanda Rinden, RD
Lois Neaton, PT
Carol L. Tappen, BA
Sadie Norby Gardner, BA
Cindy Schallock, BA

Editor/Production Manager

Jeanne Mettner,
MA, ELS, Planetary Ink
Julie Sherburne, BS, Graphic Designer

Illustrations/Design

J Campbell, Artville, Inc.

To purchase additional copies of "How did this happen?" visit the Park Nicollet Health and Care Stores at www.parknicollet.com/stores

Methodist Hospital

Eating Disorders Institute

Methodist Hospital Eating Disorders Institute provides specialized services for the primary prevention, early intervention and treatment of eating disorders, using a multidisciplinary, team-based approach across a comprehensive continuum of care, including outpatient, intensive outpatient, partial-day hospital, inpatient, and residential care settings.

Eating Disorders Institute
6490 Excelsior Boulevard
Saint Louis Park, MN, USA 55426
1-800-862-7412

http://www.parknicollet.com/edi